Acupuncture Sports Handbook

Unlocking Athletic Performance With Sports Acupuncture

Dr. Sanjay Karia

Grosvenor House
Publishing Limited

This book is published by
Grosvenor House Publishing Ltd
Link House
140 The Broadway, Tolworth, Surrey, KT6 7HT.
www.grosvenorhousepublishing.co.uk

A CIP record for this book
is available from the British Library

ISBN 978-1-80381-792-7

Disclaimer

This book, Acupuncture Sports Handbook; Unlocking Athletic Performance with Sports Acupuncture is written for trained and qualified Acupuncture practitioners of Traditional Chinese Medicine. The handbook is written in good faith, based on the experiences of the author. Practitioners who follow the techniques in this book should also use their own medical knowledge and training when treating sports and musculoskeletal injuries. The author cannot take responsibility for improper techniques, avoiding medical advice and for the need of further referral, which requires the judgement of the practitioner.

Particular attention is drawn to the chapter on Trigger Point Therapy. Trigger points are not the same as acupuncture points and the suggested trigger points should only be used by practitioners who are suitably trained and certified in Trigger Point Therapy.

Dedication

Amidst the challenges of the COVID-19 pandemic in 2020, with the restrictions and the inability to attend to patients, this book began to take shape. Over the period of nearly three years researching and writing the book, it was my wife, Nishi, whose unwavering determination and constant encouragement drove me forward. It was her encouragement through moments of struggle, that inspired the completion of this book. With deep appreciation, I dedicate this work to my wife, whose invaluable support made it all possible.

Contents

Chapter 1

Musculoskeletal System and Sports Injuries

The musculoskeletal system is a complex biological framework that provides the human body with structure, stability, and the ability to move.[1] It consists of two main parts: the *muscular system*, which includes both voluntary and involuntary muscles responsible for generating force and facilitating motion, and the *skeletal system*, comprising bones, joints, tendons and ligaments. Bones offer support, shield vital organs, and serve as attachment points for muscles, while joints allow for movement and articulation. The musculoskeletal system, in conjunction with other tissues like cartilage and synovial fluid, allows a wide range of activities, from delicate tasks to powerful movements like running and lifting.

Muscular System

The muscular system is a sophisticated organised system of muscles and related tissues that work together harmoniously, generating power, facilitating movement, maintaining posture and producing heat. It also safeguards organs, for example, the diaphragm, a dome-shaped muscle located beneath the lungs, physically protecting the lungs, where it also creates pressure differentials and protects the lungs by regulating airflow.

The muscular system comprises three types of muscles; cardiac, smooth and skeletal. Cardiac muscles are exclusively located in the heart and have distinctive characteristics enabling them to contract continuously, flexibly and efficiently. Smooth muscles, also called involuntary muscles, are found in the walls of internal organs such as the digestive system, blood vessels, and respiratory passages. They are responsible for involuntary movements, such as the contraction of the stomach during digestion or the narrowing of blood vessels. Both smooth and cardiac muscles are not under conscious control. These two muscle types are not discussed.

Muscles – Skeletal System

Most sources estimate that over six hundred and fifty skeletal muscles are found in the human body, causing a wide range of movements such as flexion, extension, abduction and adduction.[2]

Skeletal muscles, also known as voluntary or striated muscles, are a type of muscle tissue responsible for movement in the body. They are characterised by their striped or striated appearance due to the organisation of the contractile proteins, actin and myosin within the muscle fibres. Skeletal muscles, attached to bones via tendons, contract when stimulated by nerve impulses, generating force and causing joint movement. Skeletal muscles work in pairs or groups to produce coordinated movements. When one muscle contracts, its counterpart, the antagonist muscle, relaxes to allow the desired movement. For example, the biceps and triceps muscles in the upper arm work together to flex and extend the elbow joint.

Role of the Somatic Nervous System

The somatic nervous system, which is part of the peripheral nervous system, initiates and controls the actions of the body, controlling voluntary movements and carrying sensory information from the body's sensory organs to the central nervous system (CNS).[3] It coordinates voluntary muscle actions and transmits sensations like touch, pain, temperature, and proprioception (awareness of body position) to the brain for interpretation.

The somatic nervous system contains two major types of neurons, sensory neurons, which carry impulses to the central nervous system and motor neurons, which transmit impulses from the CNS, connecting to the muscles via a neuromuscular system of junctions called motor endplates. When a nerve impulse arrives at the motor end plate, the impulse causes a release of neurotransmitters such as acetylcholine, which form a bridge at the intersection, enabling the nerve impulse to travel to the muscle fibre, causing it to contract by a theory called *sliding filament theory*.[4]

Voluntary Movement

For convenience, the process of voluntary movement can be categorised into three main stages: *planning, initiation, and execution*, each with specific processes and brain involvement.

- During the *planning stage*, the motor cortex, located in the brain's frontal lobe, integrates various inputs to develop a motor plan. This includes environmental cues, task requirements, and previous experiences. The motor cortex also integrates sensory information, memories, and goals to generate an optimised motor plan. It coordinates with other brain regions, such as the basal ganglia and cerebellum, for appropriate movement selection, sequencing, and coordination.

- Moving on to the *initiation stage*, the motor plan formulated in the motor cortex is converted into neural signals that can be transmitted to the muscles.[5] The motor cortex sends signals, known as action potentials, through the corticospinal tracts, which extend from the brainstem to the spinal cord. Upper motor neurons in the motor cortex generate action potentials that travel down these tracts to reach the lower motor neurons in the spinal cord.[6] The signals undergo refinement and modulation within the brainstem to ensure precise timing, coordination, and movement control.

- Finally, in the *execution stage*, the motor signals transmitted from the lower motor neurons in the spinal cord reach the muscles. Motor neurons deliver these signals to the muscles, which directly innervate the skeletal muscle fibres via the neuromuscular junctions. At the neuromuscular junction, neurotransmitters like acetylcholine are released. These neurotransmitters bind to receptors on the muscle fibres initiating a cascade of events that lead to muscle contractions. The coordinated action of various muscles, including agonist-antagonist pairs and synergistic muscle groups, work together to produce the intended movement.

Throughout the execution of movement, sensory feedback from proprioceptors and other sensory receptors informs the brain about the ongoing movement. This constant sensory feedback to the brain allows modifications to the motor plan, initiation, or execution as needed. This feedback is crucial as it allows for real-time adjustments and corrections to ensure accurate and required movement.

The planning, initiation, and execution stages are intricately connected, occurring rapidly and seamlessly during voluntary movement. The integration and coordination of these stages involving the motor cortex, basal ganglia, cerebellum, brainstem, and spinal cord, work in harmony to enable the person to perform a wide range of voluntary movements with control and precision.

Sometimes there is confusion between voluntary movement described above and involuntary movement. Involuntary

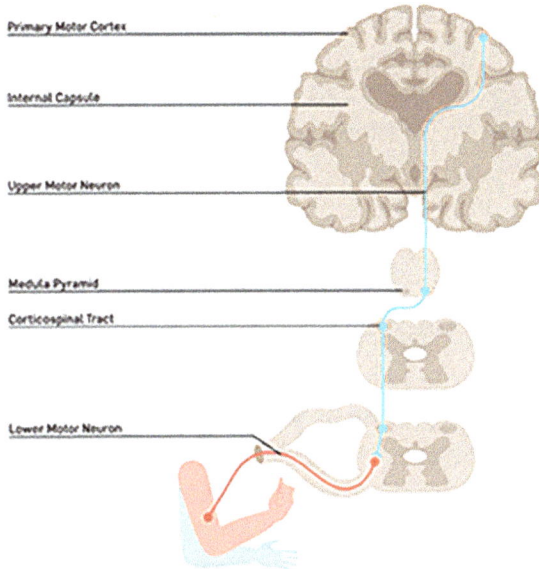

Primary Motor Cortex

Internal Capsule

Upper Motor Neuron

Medulla Pyramid

Corticospinal Tract

Lower Motor Neuron

Pyramidal Tract

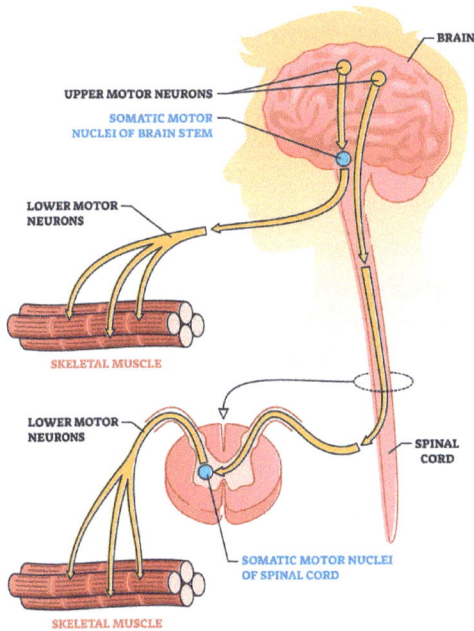

BRAIN

UPPER MOTOR NEURONS

SOMATIC MOTOR
NUCLEI OF BRAIN STEM

LOWER MOTOR
NEURONS

SKELETAL MUSCLE

LOWER MOTOR
NEURONS

SPINAL
CORD

SOMATIC MOTOR NUCLEI
OF SPINAL CORD

SKELETAL MUSCLE

Somatic Nervous System

movement is an automatic and involuntary response to a specific stimulus, bypassing conscious thought and aimed at protecting the body from harm – consisting of a reflex arc. Voluntary movement, in contrast, is a purposeful and conscious action initiated and managed by the brain, involving planning and coordination.

Structure of Muscles

Depending on the type of skeletal muscle, each muscle comprises thousands of muscle fibres wrapped together by connective tissue sheaths. Individual bundles of muscle fibres are known as fasciculi (plural fasciculus). Each muscle fibre comprises repeating units of sarcomeres, the basic functional unit of the skeletal muscle. Thousands of sarcomeres can be within a single muscle cell, depending on the muscle. The sarcomere contains, amongst other cellular components, protein fibres, actin (thin) and myosin (thick). When the nerve impulse reaches the sarcomere, as described above, an action potential causes the protein fibres to slide past each (sliding filament theory). The collective shortening of the sarcomeres along the length of the muscle fibre causes the muscle to contract, creating movement. This force is transmitted via the tendons causing movement at the joint.

The outermost connective tissue wrapping the entire muscle is known as the epimysium. The connective tissue sheath covering each fasciculus is known as perimysium, and the innermost sheath surrounding individual muscle fibre is known as endomysium.[7] The epimysium, perimysium and endomysium extend beyond the fleshy part of the muscle, and fascia and other connective tissue become thicker and collagenous, forming a tendon. Tendons attach to the periosteum of the bone at junctions called osteotendinous junctions. Tendons transmit contractile forces from the muscle to the bone, creating movements such as flexion and extension.

The proximal (end) attachment of the tendon is called the origin, and the distal end of the tendon is called the insertion.

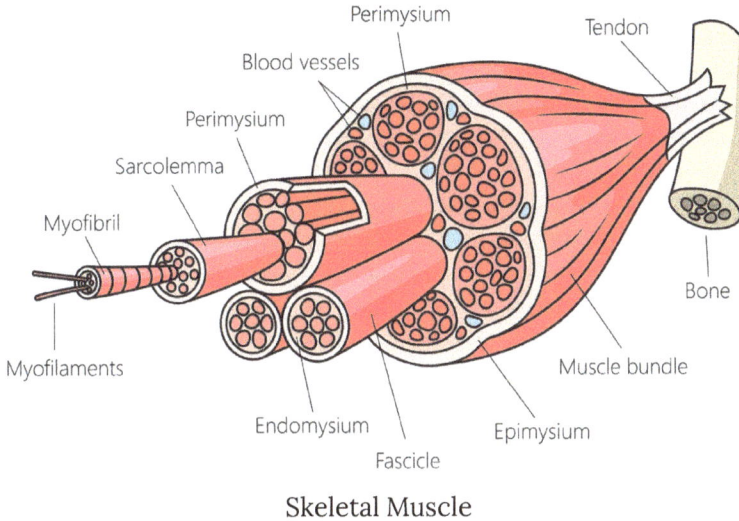

Skeletal Muscle

Muscle and Tendon Injuries – Strains

A muscle strain, also known as a pulled muscle, is a musculoskeletal injury caused by the stretching or tearing of muscle fibres due to excessive force or overuse. It commonly occurs during physical activities, sports, or movements that place undue stress on the muscles.

Signs of a muscle strain:

- Pain: Muscle strains usually result in localised pain at the injury site. The pain intensity can vary and may worsen when moving or engaging the affected muscle in specific activities.

- Muscle Weakness: Strained muscles may feel weak, making it difficult to exert normal strength. This weakness can impact the ability to perform specific movements or activities involving the injured muscle.

- Swelling: Muscle strains often lead to swelling. The injured area may appear swollen or tender to touch due to inflammation and fluid buildup.

- Muscle Spasms: Muscle strains can sometimes cause involuntary muscle contractions or spasms. These spasms can contribute to additional pain and discomfort.

- Limited Range of Motion: Strained muscles may exhibit reduced flexibility and restricted range of motion. Moving the affected muscle or joint can be challenging or painful.

- Bruising: Severe muscle strains may result in bruising or discolouration of the skin around the injury site. This occurs due to bleeding within the muscle or surrounding tissues.

- Muscle Stiffness: The affected muscle may feel stiff and tight following a muscle strain. This stiffness can further impede movement and add to the discomfort.

Grading system used for strains:

- Grade 1 (Mild): A grade 1 strain involves stretching or minor tearing of a few muscle fibres. Symptoms are generally mild and may include localised pain, minimal swelling, and minimal loss of strength or range of motion. The injured muscle may feel sore and tender, but the overall function is not significantly affected.

- Grade 2 (Moderate): A grade 2 strain indicates a more significant injury with partial tearing of comparatively larger number of muscle fibres. Symptoms are more pronounced and may include moderate pain, noticeable swelling, muscle weakness, and reduced range of motion. The affected area may be visibly bruised, and functional impairment is more apparent.

- Grade 3 (Severe): A grade 3 strain is the most severe and involves a complete tear or rupture of the muscle.[8]

This type of strain typically results in intense pain, extensive swelling, severe muscle weakness, significant loss of range of motion, and marked functional impairment.[9] There may be visible deformity or a gap in the muscle, and bruising is often prominent.

THREE GRADES OF CALF STRAIN

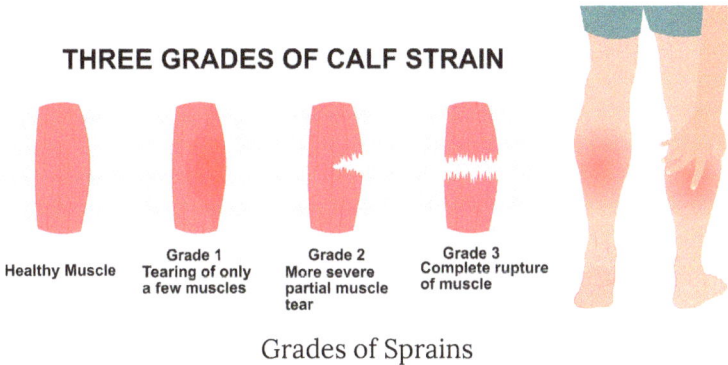

Healthy Muscle   Grade 1
Tearing of only
a few muscles

Grade 2
More severe
partial muscle
tear

Grade 3
Complete rupture
of muscle

Grades of Sprains

Tendon Injuries

Tendon injuries are known as tendonitis or tendinopathy. Tendonitis is tendon inflammation caused by overuse, repetitive movements, or injury. Tendinopathy is a broader term encompassing inflammatory and degenerative conditions affecting tendons. It involves structural changes in the tendon, resulting in pain, dysfunction, and impaired healing. Tendinopathy can be caused by chronic overuse, repetitive strain, ageing, or underlying medical conditions.

Symptoms of Tendonitis

Tendonitis can manifest in various body regions like the shoulder, elbow, wrist, hip, knee, and ankle. Specific symptoms and pain locations will depend on the particular tendon involved.

- Pain: This is the primary indicator, often described as a dull, persistent ache near the affected tendon. The pain tends to worsen with movement or activities when using the affected muscle and tendon.

- Tenderness: The region surrounding the affected tendon may be sensitive when touched.

- Swelling: Localized swelling may be present around the tendon.

- Stiffness: A feeling of rigidity, particularly noticeable in the morning or after periods of inactivity, which usually eases with gentle motion.

- Reduced Strength: A noticeable decline in muscle power or increased difficulty in tasks involving the affected muscle and tendon.

- Crepitus: In some instances, you might hear or sense a grinding or crackling sensation during tendon movement.

- Redness or Warmth: In more severe cases, there may be heightened inflammation leading to redness or warmth in the affected area.

Symptoms of Tendinopathy:

- Tendinopathy and Tendinitis are related conditions affecting tendons, but they exhibit distinct characteristics. Tendinopathy is a broader term encompassing both tendinitis (inflammation) and tendinosis which is degeneration without significant inflammation. Tendinopathy tends to be more chronic, developing gradually due to repetitive stress on the tendon. Tendinitis specifically involves inflammation of the tendon, often as a response to overuse or acute injury and is often linked to recent increased activity or strain. Pain with tendinopathy can be persistent, not solely related to activity, and may be present even at rest. Alongside pain, stiffness and weakness can also be notable features. While both conditions may share some common symptoms, the distinction lies in whether inflammation is a prominent feature (tendinitis) or if it primarily involves degeneration (tendinosis), which tends to be more chronic in nature. It is important to note that in clinical practice, the terminology can sometimes be used interchangeably.

Skeletal System

The skeletal system consists of bones and various connective tissues that collectively provide support, protection, and form to the human body. It is an essential system, functioning in multiple roles, such as facilitating movement, storing minerals, producing blood cells, and protecting internal organs.

The bones of the skeletal system provide a rigid and durable framework to support the body's structure. Through the elaborate arrangement of bones, joints, and associated connective tissues, the skeletal system ensures proper alignment and optimal distribution of weight, enabling the human body to uphold an upright posture despite the strong pull of the force of gravity. Furthermore, the skeletal system provides attachment points for muscles, tendons, and ligaments, ensuring their proper alignment and facilitating their optimal function in coordinated movements.

The skeletal system, especially the bones of the lower limb, the femur, tibia and fibula, and the bones of the foot, are structurally designed to withstand the high compressive forces associated with standing, walking, running, and jumping. For example, the curvature of the tibia, known as tibial concavity, plays a role in accommodating and dispersing the body's weight and the forces applied to it. The curvature also enhances the bone's resistance to bending and torsional stresses, supporting its capacity to endure the loads placed on it. Moreover, the slight curve in the tibia contributes to the stability of the leg and aids in shock absorption. As weight is transferred from the femur to the tibia, the curvature

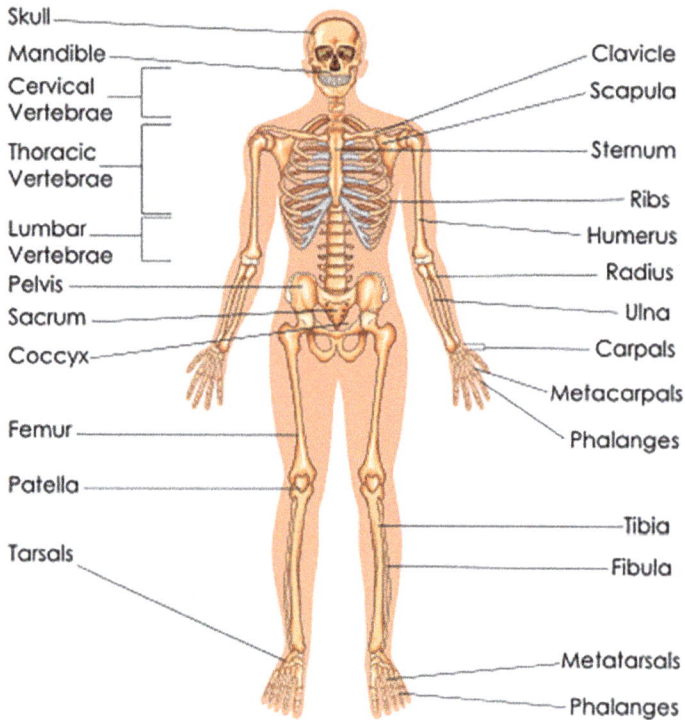

Skull
Mandible
Cervical Vertebrae
Thoracic Vertebrae
Lumbar Vertebrae
Pelvis
Sacrum
Coccyx
Femur
Patella
Tarsals

Clavicle
Scapula
Sternum
Ribs
Humerus
Radius
Ulna
Carpals
Metacarpals
Phalanges
Tibia
Fibula
Metatarsals
Phalanges

Skeletal System

helps evenly distribute and absorb forces along the length of the bone, reducing the impact on the joints and other structures of the lower limb. This mechanism promotes optimal stability and diminishes the risk of excessive stress on the surrounding tissues. The foot's structure, including its arches, bones, connective tissue, muscles, and tendons, collaboratively functions to distribute the body's weight efficiently, ensuring proper weight distribution through the feet and facilitating smooth movement during weight-bearing tasks.

Skeletal bones also provide anchor points for tendons and ligaments. Tendons are tough, fibrous connective tissues that connect muscles to bones, while ligaments are bands of connective tissue that connect bones to other bones, providing stability to joints. Tendons attach to bones at specific sites called tendon insertions or tendon attachments. They often attach to the periosteum, which is the outer layer of the bone. The strong attachment between tendons and bones allows for the transmission of forces generated by muscle contractions to the skeletal structures, enabling movement and exertion of strength.

Ligaments, on the other hand, provide stability to joints by connecting bones to other bones. They also reinforce joint capsules and help limit excessive movements that could cause injury. Ligaments are typically located at or around joints, supporting and controlling the range of motion.

The skeletal system also supports and protects internal organs and soft tissues, such as the ribcage shielding the heart, lungs, and other organs within the thoracic cavity. The vertebral column envelopes and protects the delicate spinal cord, and the skull protects the brain.

Bones also act as reservoirs for minerals and enable the regulation of mineral balance, ensuring the maintenance of bone density and facilitating essential physiological functions related to muscle activity.

Long bones and those of the pelvic region contain bone marrow, which serves as the site of haematopoiesis, which is the production of red blood cells, white blood cells, and platelets occurring within this marrow.

Ligaments and Ligament Injuries

The word ligament is derived from the Latin, "ligature", which translates to bind and tie, and this reflects the functions of ligaments. Ligaments also function to stabilise and support joints. Another essential function of ligaments is to keep and hold internal structures and organs in place. These peritoneal ligaments hold organs such as the uterus, stomach, and intestines in place by a series of ligaments.

Ligaments are composed of collagen fibres. These collagen fibres are arranged in a parallel or crisscross pattern, providing strength and stability to the ligament. The arrangement of collagen fibres varies depending on the specific ligament and its function. Elastin is a protein found in ligaments that provides some elasticity and flexibility. It allows ligaments to stretch and then return to their original shape. The precise composition of ligaments may vary depending on their location and specific function within the body. For example, ligaments in weight-bearing joints like the knee may have a higher collagen content to provide greater strength. In contrast, ligaments in a more mobile joint like the shoulder may have more elastin to increase flexibility.

Ligaments are found throughout the body but are especially prominent in and around joints, such as the knee, shoulder, ankle, and wrist. They help to maintain joint stability by preventing excessive movement or misalignment of the bones. Ligaments also aid in guiding and controlling the range of motion of joints. In addition to their role in movement, ligaments also have a sensory function as they contain receptors which provide the brain with information about the position and movement of the joint. This feedback helps with coordination, balance and joint awareness.

There are different types of ligaments in the body, including:

- Articular ligaments: Surround and stabilise joints, connecting one bone to another. They are responsible for preventing excessive movement or dislocation of the joint.

- Intracapsular ligaments: Are found inside joint capsules and help control the range of motion within the joint.

- Extracapsular ligaments: Located outside the joint capsule and provide additional reinforcement and stability.

Ligament Injury – Sprains

One of the main functions of the ligament is to make joints stable and guide joints through their normal range of motion. During movement, when a low-level load or tensile stress is applied to a ligament, this will initially manifest as non-linear stiffness. As an increasing load or tensile stress is applied, the degree of ligament stiffness increases.[10] Varying and increasing the application of the tensile force or load beyond its capacity will cause the ligament to sustain a strain injury.[11] The amount of damage is proportional to the excess stress or load applied. The greater the load or force, the more severe the sprain injury (Grade I, II and III injuries described below).

Although sprains occur when a ligament is stretched beyond its normal range, other factors, such as muscle imbalance and biomechanical abnormalities, may also contribute to sprains. Ligaments also have mechanoreceptors embedded in them. These mechanoreceptors are usually located close to the area around bone insertion, transmitting sensory and proprioceptive information about the joint position to the central nervous system.[12] With chronic injuries, these sensory receptors may get damaged and lose their sensory function, making the joint feel "loose" and more prone to increased risk of repeated sprains.

Ankle sprains are one of the most frequent injuries in athletes, so understanding the ligaments around the ankle is essential[13] (see section on ankle anatomy). Typically, ankle sprains occur when the athlete falls over and lands on the lateral side of the foot, causing a lateral ankle sprain. The three ligaments that make up the lateral complex are the anterior talofibular, the calcaneofibular and the posterior talofibular, and it is these three ligaments that tend to be injured. Although medial ankle sprains can occur, they are relatively rare due to the strong ligaments on the medial aspect of the ankle joint.

Grading of sprains

Similar to muscles strains, ligament sprains are often graded based on their severity. The grading system commonly used for sprains is as follows:

- Grade 1 (Mild): grade 1 sprain indicates a mild injury where the ligament is stretched but not torn. Symptoms include mild pain, minimal swelling, and joint stiffness or instability. The affected joint can generally bear weight and has a relatively normal range of motion.

- Grade 2 (Moderate): grade 2 sprain indicates a partial ligament tear. The injury is more significant than a grade 1 sprain and often involves noticeable pain, swelling, bruising, and joint instability. There may be some loss of function and difficulty bearing weight or performing specific movements.

- Grade 3 (Severe): grade 3 sprain signifies a complete tear or rupture of the ligament. This is the most severe type of sprain, leading to significant pain, swelling, bruising, joint instability, and loss of function. The affected joint may feel unstable, and weight-bearing or movement is usually severely limited or impossible.

The symptoms of a sprain vary based on the injury's severity; typical indications include:

- Pain: sprains commonly cause pain at the site of the injured ligament, with the intensity varying depending on the sprain's extent.

- Swelling: sprains often lead to swelling around the affected area due to the body's inflammatory response.

- Bruising: discoloration or bruising may appear near the sprained area due to blood vessel damage and bleeding.

- Limited Range of Motion: sprains can restrict the range of motion in the affected joint, making movement less comfortable and less accessible than before the injury.

- Instability: depending on the sprain's severity, joint instability or looseness may be experienced. The affected joint may feel weak or give way during use.

- Tenderness: the area surrounding the sprained ligament may be tender to the touch, with pain elicited by pressing on or near the sprained region.

- Difficulty Bearing Weight: if a weight-bearing joint, such as the ankle, is affected, putting weight on the injured limb can become challenging.

Joints

Joints are specialised anatomical structures where two or more bones meet. Their primary functions include facilitating movement, providing mechanical support, and enhancing the body's flexibility and stability.

Joints can be classified based on their structure and function.

Structural Classification:

- Fibrous Joints: Connected by dense fibrous connective tissue and allow minimal movement. Examples include sutures between skull bones and syndesmoses joints found in the lower leg between the tibia and fibula.

- Cartilaginous Joints: Connected by cartilage and allow limited movement.[14] Examples include the intervertebral discs between the spine's vertebrae and the pubic symphysis.

- Synovial joints: Also known as diarthrosis, these joints are the most widespread and adaptable type of joints present in the human body. These joints enable a broad range of motion and are characterised by a synovial cavity containing synovial fluid. The synovial fluid lubricates the joint, minimising friction and facilitating smooth movement between the connecting bones.

Key characteristics of synovial joints include:

- Articular Cartilage: the bones' joint ends are covered with smooth and slippery articular cartilage, which acts as a cushion, reducing friction during joint motion.

- Joint Capsule: surrounding the joint is a sturdy, fibrous joint capsule that encloses the joint cavity. This capsule contributes to joint stability and provides support to the bones.

- Synovial Membrane: The inner lining of the joint capsule, known as the synovial membrane, secretes synovial fluid. This fluid lubricates the joint and nourishes the articular cartilage.[15]

- Bursae: Some synovial joints have small fluid-filled sacs called bursae, situated between tendons, ligaments, and bones. Bursae act as cushions, reducing friction during movement.

Examples of synovial joints include (sub-types):

- Hinge Joint: the elbow and knee joints are hinge joints, allowing movement in a single direction, flexion and extension.

- Ball-and-Socket Joint: the shoulder and hip joints are ball-and-socket joints, enabling a wide range of motion in multiple directions.

- Pivot Joint: the joint between the neck's atlas (C1) and axis (C2) vertebrae is a pivot joint, facilitating rotational movement.

- Condyloid (Ellipsoid) Joint: the joint at the base of the fingers is a condyloid joint, allowing flexion, extension, abduction, and adduction movements.

- Saddle Joint: found at the base of the thumb the joint permits versatile movements in two planes.

- Gliding (Plane) Joints: Allow sliding or gliding movements between bones, the joints between the carpal bones in the wrist.

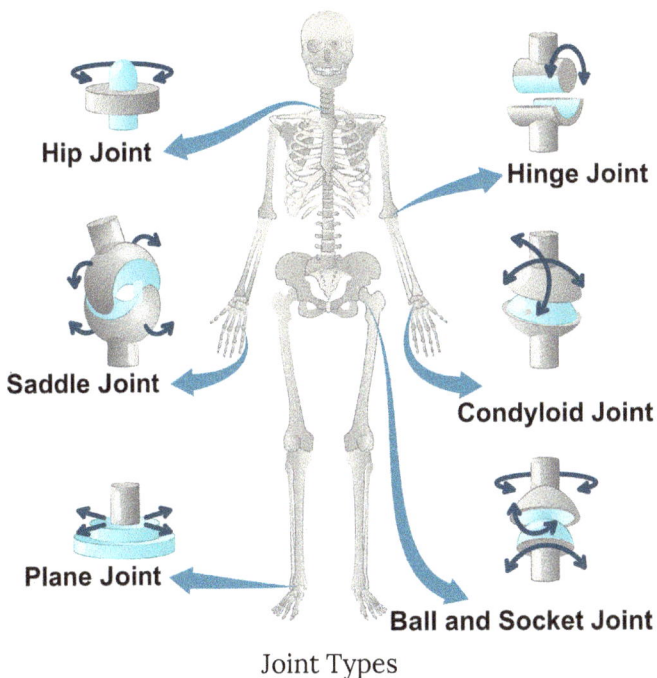

Joint Types

Functional Classification:

- Synarthroses: these joints are immovable and provide stability and protection. Fibrous and cartilaginous joints are typically classified as synarthroses.

- Amphiarthroses: these joints allow limited movement and provide some flexibility. Cartilaginous joints fall under this category.

- Diarthroses: are freely movable and allow a wide range of motions. Synovial joints belong to this category.

Conclusion

A knowledge of musculoskeletal tissues is important for understanding sports injuries. Bones, muscles, tendons, ligaments, and cartilage collectively create the body's structure and movement. Bones provide stability, muscles enable movement, tendons and ligaments connect, and cartilage cushions joints. Sports injuries often result from excessive loading, poor conditioning, or biomechanical issues, affecting these tissues. Knowledge of their structure informs prevention, treatment, and injuries from reoccurring.

References

1. Musculoskeletal System: Introduction, Anatomy/Physiology Review. www: medical-surgical-nursing/musculoskeletal review.
2. Lee, Jung P., et al. "Decellularized Tissue Matrix for Stem Cell and Tissue Engineering." Advances in Experimental Medicine and Biology, 2018.
3. Nervous System Structure & Function – MCAT Biology. Med. School Coach.
4. Nature education citation: Krans, J.L (2010) The Sliding Filament Theory of Muscle Contraction. Nature Education 3(9): 66
5. Upper motor neurons (video) | Khan Academy. www. khanacademy.org.biological-basis-of-behavior upper-motor-neurons.

6. Electrochemical Signal Amplification in Olfactory and Taste Evaluation.www:encyclopedia.pub/entry

7. Frontera WR, et al. Skeletal muscle: a brief review of structure and function. 2015 Mar;96(3):183-95

8. Can I Run With A Hamstring Strain? www.marathonhandbook.com/hamstring-strain.

9. Llinás, Adolfo, et al. "Gluteal biopolymers and aggressive synovitis of the hip joint: A news reported association. 2022

10. Woo SL et al. Biomechanics of knee ligaments. Am J Sports Med. 1999;27:533-543

11. R. Bray et al. Sports Med Arthrosc Rev 2005; 13: 127-135

12. Michelson JD, et al. Mechanoreceptors in human ankle ligaments. The Journal of Bone and Joint Surgery. Vol 77 (2): 219-224

13. Olmsted L.C., Vela L.I., Denegar C.R., Hertel J. Prophylactic ankle taping and bracing: a numbers-needed-to-treat and cost-benefit analysis. J Athl Train. 2004;39(1)

14. Load-Bearing Material Inspired by Cartilage Innovation. www.asknature.org/innovation/load-bearing-material-inspired-by-cartilage.

15. About the Knee Joint.www:bonesmart.org/knee/about-the-knee-joint/

Chapter 2

Classification and Causes of Musculoskeletal Sports Injuries

Injuries are a common occurrence in sports and activities of musculoskeletal tissues. Classifying these injuries is vital so that the practitioner can accurately diagnose, treat, and also prevent injuries from occurring in the future.

There are numerous classification systems which can be used and they have an important role in organising and categorising injuries based on specific criteria. These systems assist in identifying patterns, comparing treatment outcomes, and also developing evidence-based practices. With a structured approach to classification, the practitioner can provide more targeted and efficient care, optimising the recovery process and facilitating the athletes safe return to sports and physical activities.

Musculoskeletal and sports injuries encompass various conditions affecting the muscles, bones, joints, ligaments, tendons, and other connective tissues. These injuries can occur due to numerous factors, including trauma, overuse, repetitive stress, poor technique, inadequate conditioning, and accidents during sports or physical activities.

The Classification of Musculoskeletal and Sports injuries

- **Anatomical Classification**: This classification system categorises sports injuries based on the specific anatomical structures involved, such as muscles, bones, joints, ligaments, tendons, and other tissues. For example, a sports injury may be classified as a muscle strain, bone fracture, ligament sprain, tendonitis, or cartilage injury. This classification helps to identify the primary structures affected and guide treatment approaches specific to those structures.

- **Injury Type Classification:** Categorises sports injuries based on specific diagnoses or clinical conditions. This involves classifying injuries according to their distinct characteristics and manifestations. Examples of injury types include concussions, stress fractures, rotator cuff tears, meniscus tears, labral tears, or muscle contusions. Classifying injuries in this manner helps in understanding the nature of the injury and so providing insight into the underlying pathology.

- **Severity Classification**: Sports injuries can also be classified based on severity or grade, which helps determine the extent of tissue damage. For instance, ligament sprains are often graded as Grade I (mild), Grade II (moderate), or Grade III (severe), indicating the degree of ligament tearing or disruption. Classifying injuries with this method helps predict recovery time, plan rehabilitation protocols, and assess the need for referrals to other practitioners, such as physiotherapy and possible surgical intervention.

- **Mechanism of Injury Classification**: This classification system emphasises identifying the particular mechanism or cause of the sports injury. It categorises injuries based on how they occurred, such as contact or non-contact injuries, overuse injuries and traumatic injuries.

Understanding the mechanism of injury helps implement injury prevention strategies, identifying risk factors associated with specific sports or activities.

- **Sports-Specific Classification**: Classification based on sports or activities in which the injuries commonly occur. For instance, certain sports may have a higher prevalence of specific injuries. Examples include "runner's knee" in long-distance running, "swimmer's shoulder" in swimming, "golfer's elbow" in golf, "tennis elbow" in tennis or back problems in weight lifters. Identifying patterns and trends related to a particular sport enables targeted injury prevention strategies and preventive measures such as training modifications.

- **Time-Based Classification:** Sports injuries can be categorised based on the timing of their occurrence, distinguishing them as acute, subacute, chronic, or recurrent injuries. Acute injuries arise from a singular traumatic event, such as a sudden impact or collision. On the other hand, chronic injuries develop over time due to repetitive stress or overuse, frequently observed in sports involving repetitive motions like running or throwing. When classifying musculoskeletal and sports injuries, it is essential to consider the distinct symptoms that differentiate acute and chronic injuries. Acute symptoms arise suddenly after an injury and are characterised by intense pain at the affected site, often accompanied by swelling, inflammation, and bruising. This may lead to a limited range of motion, joint instability, and muscle spasms.

In contrast, chronic symptoms develop gradually over time and persist longer. They involve persistent pain, stiffness, tenderness, weakness, and reduced flexibility in the injured area. Additionally, individuals with chronic injuries may experience recurring episodes of discomfort, especially during increased activity.

Characteristic	Acute Injuries	Chronic Injuries
Examples	Sprains, strains and contusions.	Tendinitis, stress fractures and arthritis.
Onset	Rapid and sudden.	Gradual development over an extended period.
Cause	Often as a result of sudden accident or trauma.	Frequently linked to prolonged use or underlying condition.
Symptoms	Intense pain, swelling and bruising.	Mild to moderate pain/discomfort, stiffness and pain.
Duration	Typically short-lived, lasting days or weeks.	Extended duration, spanning weeks to months or longer.
Inflammation	Frequently accompanied by acute inflammation (with classic signs of inflammation).	Persistent inflammation, but of lower intensity.
Tissue Damage	Involves tissue damage and bleeding.	Characterised by tissue breakdown and degeneration.
Healing Time	Generally faster recovery process.	Requires more time for healing and recuperation.
Treatment Approach	Early stages: RICE (rest, ice, compression and elevation.	Addressing symptoms and root cause through treatment.
Rehabilitation	Shorter and less comprehensive rehabilitation.	More extensive rehabilitation measures.
Complications	Less likely.	Tends to result in lingering issues and challenging treatment.

Table to show differences between Acute and Chronic Injuries.

Understanding the differences between acute and chronic symptoms is crucial for accurate injury classification, as it guides appropriate treatment, rehabilitation, and preventive strategies. The diagram below summarises the differences between acute and chronic injuries.

Primary and Secondary Injuries

This classification system improves communication among healthcare providers, enhances patient understanding, and supports educational efforts in the medical field. Distinguishing primary and secondary injuries also leads to better patient outcomes and overall healthcare quality. Classifying injuries into primary and secondary categories helps prioritize treatment, prevent complications, and plan for rehabilitation. Accurate documentation can also help in cases of litigation and insurance claims, while research benefits from data analysis.

Primary injury refers to the initial damage or trauma sustained by tissues, organs, or body structures immediately following an accident or event. It is the direct result of the force or impact that occurs at the moment of injury. These acute injuries occur immediately and directly due to the traumatic event, which is typically identifiable at the time of the incident. As a consequence of primary injury, secondary injuries can develop later. Examples include sprains, strains, tendinitis, fractures and contusions.

Secondary injury is additional damage which occurs following a primary injury. Secondary injuries often result from the body's response to the primary injury as a consequence of continued trauma, lack of proper treatment or complications which may arise from the primary injury. These injuries are usually overuse and chronic in nature.

Causes of Injuries

Recognising the cause of an injury can enable the practitioner to create personalised treatment plans tailored to the individual athlete's/patient unique needs, ensuring more effective and efficient recovery. Moreover, identifying potential risk factors allows athletes and coaches to optimise performance by adjusting training programs and techniques and reducing the risk of injuries while enhancing athletic capabilities. This comprehensive approach promotes successful rehabilitation and injury prevention for athletes, improving overall sports performance and long-term well-being.

Below is a summary description of the main causes of musculoskeletal and sports injuries;

- **Intrinsic causes of injury.**

  Anatomical imbalances can contribute to the transfer of uneven forces onto joints like the ankle, knee, hip, and spine when the body is out of alignment. This imbalance affects the body's biomechanics and functioning, potentially leading to injury over time. Examples of these factors include feet that are excessively pronated or supinated, differences in limb length, knock knees (genu valgum), bow legs (genu varum), and spinal deformities like kyphosis and lordosis.

- **Physiological factors.**

  Physiological processes involves both aerobic and anaerobic respiration, which impacts movement. When muscles are fatigued, they lose the ability to generate the same power as non-fatigued muscles. This creates an imbalance between the agonist and antagonist muscles, reducing flexibility and muscle tightness. Consistently stretching muscles beyond their capacity can lead to strain injuries.

There are two basic types of muscle fibres, red and white. Red muscle fibres, also known as slow-twitch fibres, have a higher abundance of mitochondria than white muscle fibres, which are also known as fast-twitch fibres. Mitochondria are organelles responsible for producing energy through aerobic respiration. Red muscle fibres which are adapted and designed for endurance activities, rely more on aerobic metabolism, requiring a greater number of mitochondria to support sustained energy production during prolonged efforts. On the other hand, white muscle fibres, designed for explosive and powerful movements, rely predominantly on anaerobic metabolism, resulting in a lower concentration of mitochondria in these fibres. Thus, red muscle fibres with more mitochondria have the ability to contract slowly and sustain their activity for more extended periods without experiencing fatigue. In contrast, white muscle fibres with fewer capillaries, myoglobin, and mitochondria contract rapidly with significant force but for shorter durations.

- **Extrinsic causes of injury.**

Extrinsic causes of musculoskeletal and sports injuries include a range of external factors that play a role in injury occurrence. These factors are not inherent to the body but are related to the surrounding environment, equipment used, and external forces acting on the body during physical activities. Poor training techniques, such as improper form or excessive intensity, can place undue stress on muscles and joints, making them vulnerable to injury. Overtraining, without adequate rest and recovery, can lead to overuse injuries, resulting in chronic pain and decreased performance.

Unsafe, uneven, slippery, or overly hard playing surfaces can contribute to falls, collisions, and traumatic injuries. Wearing inappropriate or ill-fitted sports equipment, such as poorly cushioned shoes or inadequate protective gear, can affect body alignment and increase the risk of acute injuries. In contact sports, opponent actions, such as tackles or collisions, can lead to sudden and forceful impacts, resulting in sprains, strains, or fractures.

Environmental hazards, like obstacles or debris in sports areas, can pose unexpected risks for accidents and injuries. Weather conditions, such as extreme heat or cold, can impact an athlete's performance and influence the likelihood of injury. Moreover, the lack of proper coaching, supervision, or adherence to safety guidelines in training or sports events can also contribute to improper techniques and increase the risk of injuries.

- **Nutritional factors.**

  A balanced diet of macronutrients and micronutrients is important for optimal sports performance. Macronutrients include carbohydrates, proteins and fats. Micronutrients consist of vitamins and minerals.

  - Carbohydrate group of foods is an important fuel source for an athlete as they provide glucose for energy during aerobic respiration. Glucose is stored as glycogen in both the liver as well as muscles. Muscle glycogen is the most readily available energy source for a contracting muscle. Good sources of carbohydrates are found in whole grains, fruits, milk and yoghurt.

  - Proteins are necessary for building and repairing muscles.[1] Although proteins do not provide an immediate energy source, during prolonged activity, proteins help maintain blood glucose through gluconeogenesis. Good protein sources include lean meat, poultry, fish, eggs, dairy products, lentils and nuts.[2]

  - Fats are necessary for diet to absorb fat-soluble vitamins such as vitamins A, D, E and K. Essential fatty acids (EFA's) are compounds that the body cannot manufacture and are required from an external source in foods or as supplements. EFA's perform many essential functions such as forming part of cell membranes, synthesis of prostaglandins, joint lubrication, forming haemoglobin and nerve transmission. Good fat sources include lean meat and poultry, fish, nuts, seeds, dairy products, and olive and canola oils.

Traditional Chinese Medicine (TCM) Injury Classification

The classification approach of Traditional Chinese Medicine for musculoskeletal and sports injuries differs from that of Western Medicine. TCM adopts a holistic perspective, considering the interconnectedness of the body's energy pathways and the vital balance of Qi and Blood circulation. Each injury uniquely manifests energetic imbalances within the individual's system. TCM meticulously assess the individual's pulse, tongue, and other subtle indicators to determine the precise pattern of imbalance, crafting a personalised diagnosis.

Traditional Chinese Medicine categorizes injuries by identifying their root cause and looking beyond surface symptoms. Its preventive approach aims to maintain overall well-being and the smooth flow of Qi and Blood as well as Yin Yang balance to prevent injuries before they occur. TCM perceives injuries as an interplay of complex Qi and Blood dynamics, treating not just the injury's visible signs but also the underlying imbalances to restore the body's natural balance.

Internal and External causes of Sports and Musculoskeletal Injuries

External Pathogenic Factors

It is important to note that the pathogenic factors described below are often seen in combination. For example,

Wind-Cold or Wind-Heat, Damp-Cold, and so on. The tongue and pulse patterns are used along with other diagnostic methods, to determine a comprehensive diagnosis and treatment plan.

- **Wind** is considered one of the primary external pathogenic factors. It is associated with rapid and unpredictable changes. In TCM, Wind can disrupt the flow of Qi and Blood, leading to muscle spasms, stiffness, and joint pain.

  Tongue: The tongue body may be pale with a thin white coating. If Wind is associated with Heat, the tongue may be red with a yellow coating.

  Pulse: A Floating pulse is often associated with Wind. It may also be wiry if Wind is accompanied by Heat.

- **Cold** is associated with contraction and stagnation. Exposure to cold conditions can cause constriction of muscles and blood vessels, leading to reduced flexibility and increased risk of injuries.

  Tongue: The tongue may be pale in colour, and the coating may be thick and white.

  Pulse: The pulse is often described as slow, deep, and weak. It may also be slow and tight.

- **Dampness** is associated with heaviness and stagnation. It tends to obstruct the flow of Qi and Blood, leading to symptoms like swelling, heaviness, and a sensation of "dampness" in the affected area.

  Tongue: The tongue may appear swollen, with teeth marks on the edges. The coating is often thick, white, and greasy.

  Pulse: A Slippery pulse is commonly associated with Dampness. It may feel like a rolling pearl.

- **Heat and Fire**. These pathogenic factors are associated with inflammation and excess activity. They can cause symptoms like redness, swelling, and pain in the affected area.

Tongue: The tongue may be red, possibly with a yellow coating. In severe cases, the coating may be burnt off, leaving a red, shiny appearance.

Pulse: A Rapid pulse is indicative of Heat. It may also feel full or overflowing.

Trauma and Overexertion:

- Trauma can lead to the direct disruption of Qi and Blood flow. Depending on the severity, it can result in contusions, sprains, strains, fractures, and dislocations.

- Engaging in strenuous physical activity without proper warm-up or overexertion can lead to Qi and Blood stagnation, especially if there's a sudden stop or change in movement.

Qi and Blood Stagnation:

- Qi Stagnation: Physical trauma and emotional factors, such as stress, frustration, and suppressed emotions, can lead to Qi stagnation. Physical trauma causes Qi stagnation, where the flow of Qi is blocked or slowed down at the site of injury. This can result in pain, swelling, and localized tension. Over time, if the Qi stagnation is not addressed, it can lead to chronic pain and reduced mobility. This can manifest as muscle tension, tightness, and reduced range of motion.

- Blood Stagnation: Can result from direct trauma or prolonged constriction of blood vessels. Also, Blood circulation is closely linked to Qi flow so when flow of Qi is disrupted by physical trauma, this can lead to Blood Stasis, where the Blood becomes stagnant or pools in the injured area. Blood Stasis often manifests as bruising, dark discoloration, and the formation of blood clots. It can also contribute to pain and delayed healing. This can lead to symptoms like bruising, swelling, and sharp, stabbing pain.

In TCM, the balance between Qi and Blood is fundamental for maintaining overall health and bodily function. When Qi Stagnation occurs, it directly influences the circulation of Blood. This stagnation arises from factors like emotional stress or physical overexertion, causing a blockage in the natural flow of Qi. Qi assumes the role of a commander, propelling Blood smoothly through the body's vessels. However, when Qi becomes stagnant this leads to a decrease in Blood circulation. Consequently, Blood accumulates and congeals in specific regions, resulting in symptoms such as localized pain, swelling, and even the formation of Blood Stasis. This can manifest as sharp, fixed pain, visible bruising and swelling, a sensation of coldness in the affected area due to impaired Qi warmth, or, in severe cases, the development of palpable masses or nodules. With treatment, the primary goal is to invigorate the flow of both Qi and Blood. Specific acupuncture points and herbal formulas are selected to target both the Qi stagnation, facilitating movement of Qi and Blood

Weakness or Deficiency of Qi and Blood:

- Qi Deficiency: Chronic illnesses, poor diet, and inadequate rest can lead to Qi deficiency. Weak Qi may not provide adequate support to muscles and tendons, making them more susceptible to injuries.

- Blood Deficiency: This can result from anaemia, chronic illness, or a diet lacking in essential nutrients. Insufficient Blood can lead to weak tissues, making them more prone to injuries.

Yin-Yang Imbalance:

- Excess Yang: Overexertion, excessive sweating, or prolonged exposure to hot weather can create excess Yang in the body. This can lead to symptoms like muscle cramps, spasms, and heat-related injuries.

- Excess Yin: Prolonged exposure to cold and damp conditions or excessive consumption of cold foods and drinks can lead to excess Yin. This can cause stiffness, joint pain, and reduced mobility.

Meridian Blockages

Disruptions in the flow of Qi along specific meridians can lead to imbalances. This can result in pain and dysfunction in the corresponding areas.

Improper Posture and Movement Patterns

Incorrect posture during sports or physical activities can create imbalances in muscle engagement and distribution of force. This can lead to strain and injuries over time.

Organ Imbalance

In TCM, the balance of organ function is important for maintaining overall health and preventing injuries, including sports and musculoskeletal injuries. Each organ system in TCM is associated with specific functions, elements, and meridians and an imbalance in any of these can contribute to the development of injuries.

- **Liver** is responsible for the smooth flow of Qi and Blood throughout the body. When the Liver is in balance, it ensures proper distribution of Qi, which is essential for flexible and coordinated movement. An imbalanced

Liver, often associated with emotional stress or anger, can lead to Qi stagnation. This stagnation can result in muscle tension, reduced flexibility, and an increased risk of injuries.

- **Spleen** is responsible for transforming food into nutrients and transporting them to the rest of the body. A balanced Spleen provides the necessary nourishment for muscles, tendons, and ligaments. When the Spleen is weakened (Spleen Qi deficiency), it may lead to weak or atrophied muscles, making them more prone to injuries.

- **Kidneys** are considered the foundation of vitality in TCM and are associated with the bones, joints, and lower back. Strong Kidney Qi is essential for maintaining the structural integrity of the musculoskeletal system. When Kidney Qi is deficient, it may lead to weak bones, joints, and lower back, increasing the risk of injuries.

- **Lungs** are responsible for regulating the circulation of Qi and controlling the body's defensive Qi. Proper Lung function ensures the body's ability to protect itself from external pathogens that could lead to injuries. Weak Lung Qi may result in a compromised immune system, making a person more susceptible to injuries.

- **Heart** governs the Blood and houses the Shen (mind/spirit). A balanced Heart ensures proper Blood circulation, which is vital for nourishing the muscles and tissues. When the Heart is imbalanced, it can lead to Blood stasis or inadequate nourishment of the muscles, increasing the risk of injuries.

- **Stomach,** in TCM is responsible for receiving and digesting food. It provides the source of nutrients for the entire body. A balanced Stomach ensures that the muscles and tissues receive adequate nourishment. When the Stomach is weakened (Stomach Qi deficiency), it may lead to poor muscle tone and weak connective tissues, making them more susceptible to injuries.

- **Spleen and Kidney Yang**: The balance between the Spleen and Kidney Yang is crucial for maintaining warmth in the body. Adequate warmth is necessary for proper muscle function and preventing injuries related to cold and damp conditions.

- **Heart and Kidney Yin**: The balance between Heart and Kidney Yin helps regulate the body's moisture and nourishment. When this balance is disrupted, it can lead to conditions like dryness, which can affect the joints and muscles.

The above demonstrates the diverse classifications which TCM offers for musculoskeletal and sports injuries. Each pattern represents a unique combination of symptoms and energy imbalances in the body, enabling practitioners to tailor treatment strategies to meet individual needs and promote healing. In contrast, Western Medicine mainly concentrates on managing acute conditions through medications, physical therapy, and surgical interventions to alleviate symptoms. While effectively addressing immediate concerns, Western Medicine may not explore holistic healing and long-term rehabilitation to the extent that TCM does.

Contrastingly, Western Medicine approaches injury classification from an anatomical standpoint, pinpointing the affected structures such as bones, muscles, tendons, and ligaments. Western medicine uses standardised diagnostic criteria and cutting-edge imaging technologies to focus on precise and uniform categorisation.

Conclusion

Using a well-defined classification system allows both conventional Western Medicine and Traditional Chinese Medicine practitioners, to better understand the nature of injuries. Classification also helps identify not only the physical symptoms but also the energetic (Qi) imbalances that contribute to the injury's development and progression (TCM). This holistic perspective aids in designing comprehensive treatment plans that not only target pain relief but also promote healing, enhance recovery, and reduce the risk of recurrence.

References

1. How to Complete the Nutrition of Your Body? www:newshub feed.com/food/how-to-complete-the-nutrition-of-your-body.
2. Post-Workout Nutrition: What to Eat After a Gym Workout: www.womendisease.com/post-workout-nutrition-what-to-eat-after-a-gym-workout/

Chapter 3

Inflammation

When the body suffers from an injury, infection or other harmful stimuli, the body's natural and essential immune response is *inflammation*. Inflammation is a complex biological process that aims to protect the body and promote healing; when tissue is damaged by physical injury, pathogens (like bacteria or viruses), or toxins, the immune system triggers an inflammatory response to address the problem.

There are two main types of inflammatory reactions: acute and chronic. They differ in duration, underlying causes, and effects on the body.

Acute Inflammation

The first description of the signs of acute inflammation was provided by the Roman physician Celsus around the 1st century AD.[1] In his work "De Medicina," he outlined four fundamental indicators of inflammation. Celsus' description of these signs formed the foundation for understanding how the body responds to injuries, infections, and harmful stimuli. Although the basis remains the same, over time these concepts have been refined to provide a much deeper understanding of the process of inflammation.

Acute inflammation is the immune system's rapid and transient response to harmful stimuli, such as infections, injuries, or tissue damage. It serves as a central defence mechanism and initiates the healing process. The mechanism of acute inflammation entails intricate interactions among different cells, chemicals, and blood vessels. The process involves several stages and components, beginning with a triggering event, an injurious stimulus such as microbial infection, physical injury, chemical exposure, or autoimmune reactions.

The cardinal signs and symptoms of acute inflammation, listed below, serve as clinical indicators and valuable information for diagnosis and treatment. However, it is essential to note that not all cases of inflammation exhibit all of these signs and symptoms, and the intensity of the signs and symptoms can vary depending on the specific cause and individual factors.

- *Redness (Rubor)*: The affected area may display a reddish or flushed appearance due to increased blood flow and vasodilation in response to inflammation. This occurs as nearby blood vessels widen, allowing a greater volume of blood to flow into the area.

- *Heat (Calor)*: Inflammation can result in increased temperature in the area of the injury. This temperature elevation is due to the augmented blood flow and heightened metabolic activity associated with the inflammatory process.

- *Swelling (Tumor)*: Swelling or oedema arises due to increased vascular permeability. The blood vessels become more permeable, enabling fluid, proteins, and immune cells to leak from the bloodstream into the surrounding tissue. This fluid accumulation gives rise to swelling and the characteristic appearance associated with inflammation.

- *Pain (Dolor)*: Inflammation often induces pain, typically described as aching, throbbing, or sharp. Pain arises from the activation of pain receptors, the release of inflammatory mediators, tissue damage, and the pressure exerted on nerves caused by swelling or inflammatory exudate. The mediators which often cause pain include prostaglandins, bradykinin, and histamine

- *Loss of Function:* Although loss of function was not originally included in the four cardinal signs, it is an important feature of the inflammatory process. In some instances, acute inflammation can impede the normal function of the affected area. This can manifest as restricted mobility, diminished strength, or functional limitation. Loss of function occurs due to pain, swelling, tissue damage, or the intrusion of inflammatory exudate with normal tissue activity.

Phases of Acute Inflammation

The process of acute inflammation involves a series of complex interactions between various cells, chemicals, and blood vessels and is outlined below. However, it is essential to note that while these phases provide a general overview of the sequence of events in acute inflammation, inflammation is a complex process with overlapping stages and dynamic interactions between cells and mediators. The duration and intensity of each phase can vary depending on the specific cause and individual factors.

Vascular Phase

The vascular phase is the initial phase following a triggering event, such as an injury or infection. During the vascular stage of acute inflammation, blood vessels near the site of inflammation undergo vasodilation, widening in response to harmful stimuli. This increased blood flow, mediated by chemical signals like histamine, prostaglandins, and nitric oxide, causes redness and warmth in the affected area. Concurrently, the blood vessels become more permeable, allowing fluid, proteins, and immune cells to move from the bloodstream into the surrounding tissue, leading to swelling or oedema.

Cellular Phase

In the cellular stage, neutrophils, a type of white blood cell, participate in the inflammatory response. They undergo margination, lining up along the vessel walls, followed by rolling facilitated by interactions between adhesion molecules on the neutrophils and endothelial cells. Adhesion occurs when the neutrophils firmly attach to the vessel walls, driven by stronger binding between adhesion molecules and receptors on the endothelial cells.[2] Subsequently, the neutrophils migrate through the vessel walls and into the tissue, a process known as transmigration or diapedesis. Chemotactic factors guide the neutrophils towards the site of inflammation, ensuring they reach the specific location where their actions are needed. Once in the tissue, neutrophils engage in phagocytosis, engulfing and destroying foreign particles, such as bacteria, debris, or pathogens.[3]

Exudation Stage

The Exudation phase stage follows the cellular phase. During this phase, fluid, proteins, and immune cells are leaked from the blood vessels into the surrounding tissue. Increased vascular permeability allows plasma fluid to move from the bloodstream into the tissue, leading to fluid accumulation and the formation of inflammatory exudate. This exudate contains immune cells, including neutrophils and macrophages, as well as proteins like clotting factors and antibodies. It aids in diluting toxins, delivering immune cells and necessary components for tissue repair, and facilitating the removal of debris from the inflamed site.

Phagocytosis also occurs when immune cells, like neutrophils and macrophages, engulf and eliminate foreign particles, such as bacteria and cellular debris, within the affected tissue. Alongside phagocytosis, these immune cells release inflammatory mediators, such as cytokines, chemokines, and prostaglandins. These mediators play a crucial role in intensifying the immune response, as they not only enhance the immune activity but also attract additional immune cells to migrate towards the site of inflammation.[4]

Resolution Phase

During the resolution phase of acute inflammation, the inflammatory response gradually diminishes as the harmful stimuli are neutralised or eliminated.[5] The resolution phase encompasses several processes that work towards restoring normal tissue function and promoting healing as below;

- Dampening of Inflammatory Response: Specialised cells, such as macrophages, play a vital role in the resolution phase. They release anti-inflammatory chemicals which help suppress the immune response and reduce inflammation. This includes the production of anti-inflammatory cytokines and the clearance of inflammatory mediators.

- Clearance of Cellular Debris: Resolving macrophages and other immune cells actively participate in clearing the cellular debris that remains from the inflammatory process. They engulf and remove dead cells, pathogens, and other waste products from the inflamed tissue.

- Tissue Repair and Regeneration: The resolution phase initiates tissue repair and regeneration. Specialised cells, such as fibroblasts, become activated to produce collagen, a structural protein that aids in rebuilding and strengthening the damaged tissue. Additionally, new blood vessels form to enhance oxygen and nutrient supply to the area.

- Angiogenesis and Granulation Tissue Formation: Angiogenesis or forming new blood vessels, occurs during the resolution phase to support tissue repair. The development of granulation tissue, composed of new blood vessels, fibroblasts, and collagen, facilitates the reorganisation and restoration of the tissue structure.

- Remodelling and Scar Formation: As the resolution phase progresses, the damaged tissue undergoes remodelling. The newly formed tissue matures and reorganises to restore functionality. In some instances, scar tissue may develop as part of the healing process, providing structural support but lacking the complete functionality of the original tissue.

- Restoration of Normal Function: Ultimately, the resolution phase aims to restore the affected area to its pre-inflammatory state and regain normal tissue function. The intensity of the inflammatory response subsides, and the immune system returns to a balanced state.

Typically, the acute inflammation's response restores the tissues, however if resolution is not achieved, this can result in a chronic inflammation.

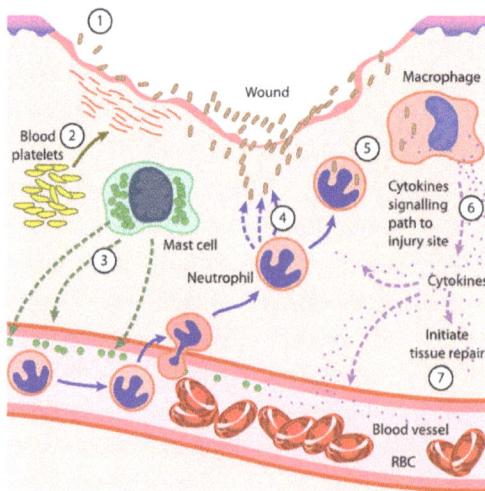

1. Bacteria and other pathogens enter wound

2. Platelets from blood release blood-clotting proteins at wound site

3. Mast cells secrete factors that mediate vasodilation and vascular constriction. Delivery of blood, plasma, and cells to injured area increases

4. Neutrophils secrete factors that kill and degrade pathogens

5. Neutrophils and macrophages remove pathogens by phagocytosis

6. Macrophages secrete hormones called cytokines that attract immune system cells to the site and activate cells involved in tissue repair

7. Inflammatory response continues until the foreign material is eliminated and the wound is repaired

Inflammation

Musculoskeletal Chronic Inflammation

Chronic inflammation in musculoskeletal injuries refers to a prolonged inflammatory response in the affected tissues, including muscles, tendons, ligaments, or joints. It can occur due to acute injuries that do not heal properly, repetitive stress, or overuse injuries. Chronic inflammation can also be associated with tendinitis, bursitis, or arthritis.

When an injury or overuse occurs, the body initiates an acute inflammatory response to repair the damaged tissues. This involves releasing immune cells and chemicals to clear debris, promote healing, and prevent infection. Usually, once the injury heals, the inflammation subsides. However, in cases where the injury is severe, repetitive, or fails to heal correctly, the inflammatory response can become chronic. Various factors contribute to the development of chronic inflammation in musculoskeletal injuries:

- **Failure of proper healing**: Insufficient or impaired healing processes can play a role in chronic inflammation. When an injury occurs, the body triggers an inflammatory response to remove damaged cells and initiate tissue repair. However, the inflammatory response can persist if the healing process is disrupted due to inadequate blood supply or compromised immune response. This leads to prolonged inflammation, contributing to chronic inflammation in the musculoskeletal tissues.

- **Repetitive stress and overuse**: Musculoskeletal injuries resulting from repetitive stress or overuse, such as tendinopathies (for example, tendinitis) or stress fractures, can contribute to chronic inflammation. These injuries arise from repeated motions or excessive strain on the affected tissues without sufficient rest and recovery time. The repetitive stress causes microtrauma and small-scale tissue damage, prompting an inflammatory response for tissue repair. However, the inflammation can become chronic if the stress continues without proper healing.

- **Prolonged tissue damage**: Severe injuries or continuous stress on the musculoskeletal tissues can lead to prolonged tissue damage. This sustained damage triggers an ongoing inflammatory response as the body attempts to repair and heal the injured area. Persistent inflammation can result in tissue degeneration and contribute to chronic inflammation in the musculoskeletal structures.

- **Autoimmune reactions**: In some instances, chronic inflammation in musculoskeletal injuries may be associated with autoimmune reactions. Autoimmune diseases occur when the immune system mistakenly targets healthy tissues as foreign or damaged, leading to inflammation and tissue destruction.[6] In autoimmune-related musculoskeletal conditions like rheumatoid arthritis, the immune system attacks the joints, causing chronic inflammation and joint damage.

Signs and Symptoms of Musculoskeletal Chronic Inflammation:

- **Persistent or Recurrent Pain**: Chronic inflammation is characterised by continuous or recurring pain that may be dull, aching, or throbbing. The pain can persist even during rest and may worsen with specific movements or activities.

- **Swelling**: Chronic inflammation can cause a low-level or fluctuating swelling that persists over time. Although not as pronounced as acute inflammation, it can contribute to discomfort and hinder normal function.

- **Stiffness and Limited Mobility**: Prolonged inflammation can result in joint stiffness and reduced range of motion.[7] The affected joint or muscle may feel tight, and movement can be accompanied by discomfort or pain.

- **Weakness**: Ongoing inflammation and tissue damage can lead to muscular weakness or fatigue, reducing strength and endurance.

- **Functional Impairment**: Chronic inflammation can impact daily activities, sports performance, or occupational tasks due to pain and decreased mobility affecting overall function.

- **Tenderness**: The affected area may be tender to the touch, indicating ongoing inflammation and tissue sensitivity.

- **Structural Changes**: Long-lasting inflammation can cause structural alterations in the tissues. For instance, tendons may thicken (tendinopathy) or undergo degenerative changes, joints may experience degeneration (osteoarthritis), or bone spurs may form.

Traditional Chinese Medicine and Inflammation

In Traditional Chinese Medicine, the concept of inflammation is not explicitly described in the same way as in Western medicine. While TCM does not differentiate between acute and chronic inflammation in the same manner as Western Medicine, it does recognise patterns of excess heat, stagnation, or dampness that may manifest as symptoms similar to inflammation. However, in TCM, patterns of disharmony and imbalance in the body can be associated with symptoms resembling inflammation, as explained below.

First Stage

From a TCM perspective, traumatic injury forces the nourishing Blood out of vessels where it combines with the defensive Wei Qi, which resides typically and spreads between the skin and the muscles. When the warm and turbid Wei Qi combines with the errant nourishing Blood, the warmth of the Wei Qi "cooks" the Blood, producing a heat toxin – Xie. Xie, by nature, is evil and pathogenic Qi. The Xie heat toxin produced is due to Blood and Wei Qi not being in their proper place, so in these circumstances, both do not have the right relationship with each other. The resulting pathological change in the tissue exhibits the classic signs of inflammation described above, heat, redness, pain and swelling.

Furthermore, at the site of tissue injury, the smooth flow of Qi is disrupted as the compressive forces caused by the traumatic event damage the vessels and meridians in which Qi and Blood flow. When Qi is not flowing, Blood will also not flow, causing Blood Stasis or Blood Stagnation. This is the beginning of toxin formation and Blood Stasis.

The TCM treatment principle for the first stage described above is to primarily *clear heat, relieve pain, dispel stasis, and resolve toxins.*

The Second Stage

During the second stage of the inflammatory process, when the initial inflammation subsides, Blood Stagnation and congestion of Qi and fluids remain in the local area. This congested state causes stiffness and pain. The damaged tissue also weakens the body's defence against invading external pathogens such as Wind and Damp.

The treatment strategy for the second stage is to move Blood and dispel Stasis. Clearing Heat now becomes secondary to moving Blood and dispelling stasis. Treatment during this stage aims to decrease pain and clear the way for tissue regeneration that characterises stage three. Dispelling Blood Stasis improves the Nutritive or Ying Qi to flow better, which helps with the healing process.

Tissue damaged during injury is weak and susceptible to invasion from external evils such as Wind, Cold and Damp. Although the primary aim of treatment in the second stage is to move Blood and dispel Stasis, consideration should always be given to the presence of external evils, which, if left untreated, can cause the injury to become chronic Bi. If external evils are present (symptoms of Wind, Damp, Cold and Heat.), acupuncture points should also be used to expel and resolve the pathogens.

Third Stage

The third stage of trauma in TCM is the need to rebuild the damaged and traumatised tissue as well as protection from exogenic evils Wind, Cold and Damp. At this stage, lingering pain may be indicative of residual Blood Stasis. The five transporting points play a crucial role in treating Bi syndrome. The three transporting points along the channels distal to the elbows and knees are particularly important during treatment. The Shu Stream point is effective in enhancing Defensive Qi. The Jing River point prevents pathogenic factors from invading the joints and sinews. Using the Luo Connecting point is also effective, keeping muscles and sinews from being affected.

Key TCM Concepts and Explanations Related to Chronic Inflammation

Qi and Blood Flow Disruption

For ideal health Qi and Blood needs to flow harmoniously. Chronic inflammation arises when this flow encounters obstructions or stagnation. Stagnation of Qi and Blood can lead to accumulation of Heat and toxins, creating an environment conducive to chronic inflammatory conditions. Trauma, poor lifestyle habits, emotional disturbances, or other imbalances within the body can cause stagnation.

Accumulation of Excess Heat and Dampness

According to TCM chronic inflammation is an accumulation of excess Heat within the body, which shows as symptoms of redness, warmth, and swelling. Additionally, excess Dampness, indicating fluid retention and heaviness, can exacerbate the chronic inflammatory state. The coexistence of excess Heat and Dampness creates ideal conditions for inflammation to persist.

Deficiencies and Impaired Immune Response

With deficiencies in Qi, Blood, Yin and Yang imbalance, these states can contribute to chronic inflammation. A weakened immune system due to deficiencies can result in improper regulation of the body's inflammatory responses, allowing chronic inflammation to persist.

Organ System Imbalances

Organ imbalances can impact the body's ability to heal and recover from various health conditions. When there are imbalances, this hinders the body's natural healing processes. Organ imbalance results in;

- Disrupted flow of Qi, resulting in stagnation, blockages, or deficiencies. This can slow down the healing process and contribute to discomfort or pain.

- Inadequate nutrient supply. The Spleen is responsible for transforming food into Qi and Blood, which nourishes the body's organs and tissues. If there is an imbalance in the Spleen and Stomach system, nutrient absorption and distribution is compromised. This can lead to impaired nourishment for the body's healing processes and slowing down recovery.

- The Lungs and Kidneys functions in supporting the body's immune function. Imbalances in these organ systems can weaken the immune response, making the body more susceptible to infections and delaying the healing process. A weakened immune system might also fail to adequately control inflammation, impairing the body's healing mechanisms.

Emotional Imbalance

In TCM, emotions exert significant influence over the body's healing mechanisms. Emotions are dynamic forces that can either support or disrupt the body's internal balance. Positive emotions are associated with a smooth flow of Qi, promoting healing, while negative emotions can create imbalances that hinder the body's inherent healing capabilities. Excessive anger, for instance, can disturb the Liver's Qi flow, leading to inflammation, whereas chronic worry may interfere with the Spleen's function. Additionally, emotional stress triggers the release of stress hormones, which can affect inflammation and undermine immune responses.

Imbalance of Yin and Yang and Inflammation

An overall imbalance between Yin and Yang in the body can disrupt the harmonious functioning of the body's systems, including those involved in inflammation regulation. For instance, if there is excessive Yang energy and deficient Yin energy, it can create a Yin-Yang imbalance that favours inflammation. The excessive Yang energy generates heat and activity, while the deficient Yin energy fails to provide the cooling and nourishing qualities necessary to maintain balance. This imbalance can contribute to the manifestation of inflammatory symptoms.

Also, when there is an excess of Yang energy in the body, it can lead to symptoms of inflammation, such as redness, swelling, heat sensations, and pain. This excess Yang can result from various factors, including emotional stress, overexertion, or the accumulation of excessive Yang energy from external or internal sources. Excessive Yang energy can create an imbalance and disrupt the body's equilibrium, leading to inflammatory responses.

Yin energy represents the body's cooling, nourishing, and moistening. When Yin energy is deficient, these nourishing and cooling qualities are lacking, which can result in excess Yang energy (empty Heat). Without the balancing effect of Yin, excessive Yang can manifest as symptoms of inflammation. Yin deficiency may be caused by chronic stress, inadequate rest, poor diet, or imbalances in bodily fluids. The insufficient Yin energy fails to counterbalance Yang's Heat and activity, leading to relative excess and inflammation.

Bi Syndrome and Chronic Inflammation

The term "Bi" signifies blockage or obstruction, caused by an invasion of external Wind, Cold or Dampness, where the flow of Qi and so Blood encounters obstacles along the body's meridians, causing a category of disorders characterized by discomfort, pain, and stiffness affecting the muscles, joints, tendons, and bones. Stagnant Qi and accumulated Heat can lead to localized inflammation. The body's attempts to restore proper Qi flow and dissipate excess heat can unintentionally fuel the inflammatory processes, resulting in chronic inflammation over time.

Bi Syndrome also disrupts the smooth flow of Qi along the meridians. Meridian disruptions impede the body's ability to regulate Qi and Blood flow. This interruption may lead to localized inflammation as the body attempts to restore natural flow of Qi. If meridian disruptions persist, inflammation might become chronic due to the ongoing blockages.

Symptoms of Bi Syndrome

Symptoms of Bi Syndrome can vary but typically encompass joint pain, stiffness, restricted movement, and sensations of numbness or heaviness in the affected regions. Weather changes, especially dampness or cold conditions, can exacerbate the pain.

- Joint discomfort, pain and Stiffness is the characteristic sign of Bi Syndrome. The pain can range from sharp to dull, while stiffness is most prominent during the morning or after periods of rest.

- The affected joints typically have restricted flexibility and reduced range of motion, leading to difficulties in performing regular activities.

- With Bi Syndrome the patient might have a feeling of heaviness or numbness in the afflicted areas.

- Pain linked to Bi Syndrome is recognized for its tendency to migrate from one joint or area to another, especially if the pathogen causing Bi, is Wind.

- Symptoms of Bi Syndrome can worsen when joints are exposed to cold, damp, or humid environments. However, the symptoms of Bi Syndrome may be relieved by movement and application of warmth. Gentle physical activity and warm compresses prove beneficial.

- Affected regions maybe tender when touched, and pressure or palpation can trigger sensations of pain and discomfort.

- With Bi Syndrome, the person may feel fatigued due to the persistent discomfort and pain experienced.

- Discomfort and pain associated with Bi Syndrome often disturb sleep patterns and hinder the ability to find a comfortable sleeping position.

It is worth noting that while Bi Syndrome itself is not a direct cause of chronic inflammation, it can contribute to a state where chronic inflammation might develop. However, chronic Bi Syndrome strains the immune system, leading to reduced responsiveness. An impaired immune system may struggle to effectively manage inflammation, allowing it to persist and possibly evolve into a chronic state.

Conclusion

The inflammatory process is a sophisticated and intricate biological reaction that helps as a vital defence mechanism against harmful stimuli. This intricate response involves complex interactions among immune cells and tissues, all working together to neutralize threats and promote tissue recovery. While acute inflammation acts as a protective shield to oppose initial injuries or infections, the persistence presence of chronic inflammation can lead to a spectrum of health challenges, encompassing autoimmune disorders, cardiovascular complications, and potentially even cancer.

References

1. www.ncbi.nlm.nih.gov/books.
2. Dalakas, Marinos C. "Immunotherapy of Myositis: Issues, Concerns and Future Prospects." Nature Reviews Rheumatology, 2010.
3. How Does Macrophages Look Under Microscope? Uncovering the Secrets of the Cell. www:alloptica.com/how-does-macrophages-look-under-microscope.
4. Chen, Y., Zhang, Y., Zhao, G., Chen, C., Yang, P., Ye, S., & Tan, X. (2016). Difference in Leukocyte Composition between Women before and after Menopausal Age, and Distinct Sexual Dimorphism.
5. Inflammation Part 3: Resolving inflammation – resolvins, protectins, maresins and lipoxins. www:anti-agingfirewalls.com
6. Attack Of The Autoimmune Disease. (2014). Alternative Medicine.
7. Effect of Age-Related Musculoskeletal Conditions on Senior Golfer Physical Capacity, Golf Performance Ability and Playing Characteristics. Published in International Journal of Golf Science.

Chapter 4

Pain – Western Medicine Perspective

With musculoskeletal and sports injuries, pain is one of the most common and prominent symptoms experienced by patients. Although unpleasant, its significance lies in the fact that it serves as a crucial indicator, providing essential information to the practitioner. By understanding the characteristics and nuances of the pain, the practitioner can gain valuable information to evaluate pain as a presenting symptom and also allow the practitioner to gauge the effectiveness of the treatment and make informed decisions about further interventions.

Summary of usefulness of evaluating pain in a patient

- Making a diagnosis by understanding the location, intensity, and quality of pain, the practitioner can make a more accurate diagnosis and determine the underlying cause of the injury. This helps influence appropriate treatment strategies.

- The level of pain experienced can provide insights into the severity of the injury, indicating the extent of tissue damage and assessing potential complications when planning and treating pain.

- The assessment of pain assists the practitioner in formulating an effective treatment plan. Different injuries may require varying approaches, such as rest, physical therapy, medication, or surgical referral. In TCM, this assessment will facilitate the choice of acupuncture points to be used and the type of points, such as local, adjacent or distal.

- The pain level assists with monitoring treatment progress, as pain sensation may decrease or remain the same. Monitoring changes in pain allows the practitioner to evaluate the effectiveness of treatment and make appropriate adjustments if needed.

- Pain management is a critical component of rehabilitation and recovery. Understanding pain helps implement strategies to control and alleviate pain, allowing athletes to regain function, restore mobility, and safely return to their sport.

- Sports injuries can have significant psychological effects on the athlete, including fear, anxiety, frustration, or depression. Understanding and addressing pain appropriately can help mitigate these psychological challenges, promoting overall well-being and supporting mental recovery.

- Preventing injuries in the future. By recognising the early warning signs of pain or discomfort, athletes and their coaches can take appropriate measures to modify training techniques, prevent overuse injuries, and promote proper rest and recovery.

Types of Pain

Acute Pain

Acute pain arises suddenly and is typically related to a specific event, such as an injury or trauma. Acute pain is temporary and localised to the site of the injury, lasting for a short period of time but can last for several days or weeks, subsiding once the injury heals. The sharp sensation of pain experienced is the body's protective mechanism by alerting the individual to take action to prevent further harm.

General signs and symptoms of Acute Pain:

- Sudden onset.
- Sharp, stabbing and intense sensation.
- Feeling of restlessness or anxiety.
- Patients experiencing acute pain might instinctively guard or protect the affected area by avoiding movement or applying pressure to it.
- Limited range of motion.
- Fluctuating intensity of pain.
- Local swelling and redness.
- Sweating and pallor.
- Disturbed sleep.
- Emotional distress, causing anxiety, frustration, and irritability.

Acute pain from an injury may evolve into chronic pain if the injury does not heal or the pain pathways malfunction.

Chronic Pain

Chronic pain is persistent and long-lasting, which continues beyond the normal healing time for an injury or illness. It is generally defined as pain lasting at least three months or longer.[1] Chronic pain may also be intermittent in nature. Unlike acute pain, which is triggered by a specific event, chronic pain may lack a clear causative identifiable event. Chronic pain is often described as dull, achy with a lingering sensation and can be intermittent. Stiffness may also be present. Chronic pain can often lead to other symptoms and conditions, such as depression, anxiety and insomnia.

Chronic pain is characterized by its persistence over an extended period, typically beyond the normal time taken for tissue healing.

Chronic pain arises from a diverse range of underlying causes:

- **Inflammatory Conditions:** Chronic pain can be a consequence of inflammatory disorders like rheumatoid arthritis, osteoarthritis, and autoimmune conditions. These conditions involve persistent inflammation, leading to ongoing discomfort and joint damage.

- **Neuropathic Conditions:** Neuropathy, diabetic neuropathy, and post-herpetic neuralgia are examples of disorders that lead to chronic pain. These conditions stem from damage or dysfunction of the nervous system, resulting in sensations of burning, tingling, or shooting pain.

- **Musculoskeletal Issues:** Chronic pain often arises from problems affecting the musculoskeletal system, including fibromyalgia, myofascial pain syndrome, and chronic back pain. These conditions involve persistent pain in muscles, tendons, ligaments, and bones.

- **Injuries and Trauma:** Severe injuries, surgeries, or accidents can lead to chronic pain, especially when nerve tissues are damaged. Conditions like complex regional pain syndrome (CRPS) can develop from such trauma.

Complex Regional Pain Syndrome (CRPS) is a chronic and often debilitating condition that typically affects a limb, such as an arm or a leg. It is characterized by severe, continuous pain that is disproportionate to the initial injury. Common symptoms include changes in skin colour and temperature, swelling, sensitivity to touch, and muscle weakness. CRPS can develop after an injury or trauma, and its exact cause is not fully understood. There are two types: Type I, which occurs without direct nerve damage, and Type II, which follows a specific nerve injury. Complex regional pain syndrome and certain types of headaches involve central sensitization, which is an abnormal response of the central nervous system to pain stimuli. This leads to heightened pain sensitivity and persistent discomfort.

COMPLEX REGIONAL PAIN SYNDROME

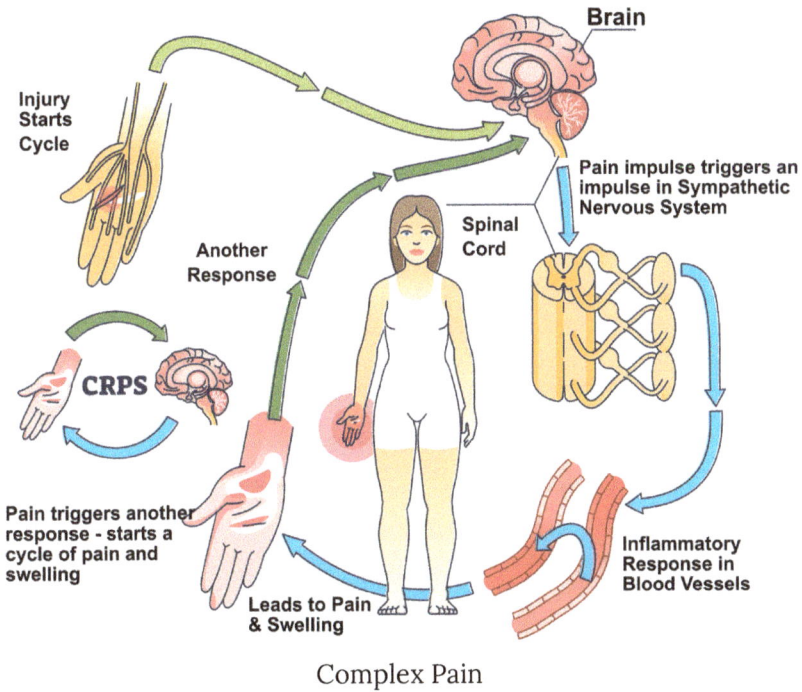

Brain

Injury Starts Cycle

Pain impulse triggers an impulse in Sympathetic Nervous System

Spinal Cord

Another Response

CRPS

Pain triggers another response - starts a cycle of pain and swelling

Inflammatory Response in Blood Vessels

Leads to Pain & Swelling

Complex Pain

- **Degenerative Conditions:** Chronic pain can result from degenerative conditions like degenerative disc disease, spinal stenosis, and spondylosis. These involve the progressive deterioration of spinal structures, leading to ongoing pain.

- **Psychological Factors:** Emotional factors like stress, anxiety, depression, and trauma can significantly influence chronic pain. These psychological elements can exacerbate or contribute to the experience of pain.

- **Visceral Pain:** Conditions like irritable bowel syndrome, endometriosis, or interstitial cystitis can lead to chronic visceral pain originating from internal organs.

- **Chronic Headaches and Migraines:** Tension-type headaches, migraines, and cluster headaches are examples of conditions that result in recurring, chronic head pain.

- **Cancer and Cancer Treatments:** Cancer-related pain can persist even after successful treatment. Additionally, treatments like chemotherapy, radiation, and surgeries can cause long-term pain.

- **Autoimmune Disorders:** Chronic pain can be associated with autoimmune disorders such as lupus, multiple sclerosis, and Crohn's disease. These conditions involve the body's immune system mistakenly attacking its own tissues.

- **Idiopathic or Unknown Causes:** In certain cases, the specific origin of chronic pain may remain unclear.

Common Signs and Symptoms of Chronic Pain

The signs and symptoms of chronic pain can vary widely depending on the underlying cause and other individual factors. Chronic pain is a complex condition that can have a significant impact on a person's physical and emotional well-being.

- Chronic pain lasts for weeks, months, or in some cases even years, often well beyond the expected recovery time for the initial injury or condition.

- Unlike acute pain, chronic pain tends to be a constant or recurrent sensation rather than one triggered by a specific event or movement.

- Chronic pain is often described as a dull, aching, burning, or throbbing sensation. It may not be as sharp or intense as acute pain.

- Patients with chronic pain may experience a reduced ability to perform daily activities, work, exercise, or even socialize due to pain-related limitations.

- Chronic pain can lead to fatigue and sleep disturbances due to discomfort and difficulty finding a comfortable position for sleep.

- Chronic pain can be associated with emotional distress, including symptoms of depression, anxiety, irritability, and frustration.

- Some patients with chronic pain may experience changes in appetite, leading to weight loss or weight gain.

- Due to the limitations caused by chronic pain, individuals might withdraw from social activities and feel isolated.

- Chronic pain can lead to hyperalgesia, which is an increased sensitivity to pain so that even a mild stimulus can result in heightened pain perception.

- With chronic pain, sensitization may occur. This is a sensation of pain which continues even after the initial cause has healed.

- Chronic pain can affect cognitive function, making it difficult to concentrate, remember things, and make decisions.

- Some patients with chronic pain may have become dependent or addicted to pain medication. If this is the case, the TCM practitioner would be advised to contact the patient's doctor so that the medical practitioner can make adjustment to the dosage as the TCM treatment take place

Other Types of Pain

- **Neuropathic pain** is usually chronic and arises from dysfunction or damage to the nervous system. The affected nerves send abnormal signals to the brain, and there is a perception of pain, even in the absence of injury or any physical damage. The sensation associated with neuropathic pain is often described as a shooting, stabbing, or burning like sensation and may have accompanying sensations of tingling, pins and needles. Like chronic pain, neuropathic pain may also be intermittent. Mobility may also be affected by neuropathic pain.

- Systemic conditions such as diabetes, multiple sclerosis and trigeminal neuralgia can cause neuropathic pain. Physical causes such as herniated discs and spinal nerve compression can give rise to neuropathic pain.

- **Nociceptive pain** is a type of pain which occurs as a result of activation of specialised nerve fibres called nociceptors. Nociceptors are specialised sensory nerve endings throughout the body, especially in the skin, muscles, joints, and internal organs. These receptors detect and transmit signals related to tissue damage such as sprains and strains. When stimulated, nociceptors send signals to the brain via the spinal cord, resulting in pain perception.

- There are two main types of pain associated with nociceptors: somatic and visceral. Somatic pain arises from activating nociceptors in the skin, muscles, bones, joints, and connective tissues. Visceral pain originates from the activation of nociceptors in the internal organs. With visceral pain, the sensation is often described as a deep, cramping, or squeezing sensation.

- **Radicular pain** is characterised by specificity and occurs when the spinal nerve undergoes compression or inflammation. Typically, the symptoms of radicular pain arise from nerve compression, which is commonly associated with disc herniation, and is mainly observed in young athletes. In more mature athletes, symptoms may arise from degenerative changes.

- Since the nerve fibres of a spinal nerve root supply sensation and strength to a particular body region, the compressed nerve will lead to symptoms in the corresponding area where the nerve provides sensation and strength. Consequently, nerves in the neck region are responsible for sensation and strength in the arms, while nerves in the lower back govern sensation and strength in the legs. These regions can also be affected by radicular pain.

- **Visceral pain** originates from internal organs and is often described as deep, dull, or squeezing. Examples include, abdominal pain from gastrointestinal disorders, pelvic pain from reproductive organ conditions.

- **Referred pain** is perceived in a different location than the actual source of the pain. Example of referred pain includes myocardial infarction pain being felt in the arm or jaw due to the shared nerve pathways between the heart and these areas.

- **Psychogenic pain** is experienced due to psychological factors. It can be just as distressing as physical pain. Stress, anxiety, depression, or underlying psychological conditions are examples.

- **Inflammatory pain** is linked to inflammation in the body and often accompanies conditions like autoimmune disorders such as rheumatoid arthritis, Crohn's disease, or other inflammatory conditions.

- **Breakthrough pain** is a sudden and intense flare-up of pain that occurs despite a person being on regular pain medication. Occurs commonly in individuals with chronic pain conditions, it can be triggered by certain activities or movements.

- **Phantom pain** is experienced in a body part that has been amputated. It's thought to arise from the brain's continued perception of the missing limb.

- **Psychosomatic pain** is influenced by psychological factors, and it can manifest as real physical pain, even when there is no apparent physical cause.

Pain Pathway

The pain pathway, sometimes called the nociceptive pathway or spinothalamic pathway, consists of multiple stages through which pain signals travel from the site of injury to the brain, where they are perceived and interpreted.

The key stages of the pain pathway include:

- **Transduction:** In this initial phase, the process begins with nociceptors activation. Certain chemicals are released at the injury site when tissue damage or injury occurs. When these stimuli exceed a certain threshold, nociceptors generate electrical signals called action potentials.

- **Transmission:** The generated action potentials are transmitted along peripheral nerve fibres towards the spinal cord. Two types of nerve fibres are involved in transmitting the stimuli; a-delta, which are myelinated nerve fibres that transmit fast, sharp, and localised pain signals. They are responsible for the initial acute pain sensation. C-fibres, on the other hand, are unmyelinated nerve fibres that transmit slower, dull, and diffuse pain signals.[2] They are responsible for the prolonged burning or aching pain sensation. The action potentials generated by the nociceptor travel along the peripheral nerve fibres via the dorsal root ganglia of the spinal cord, where they interact with excitatory and inhibitory interneurons.

- **Modulation in the Spinal Cord:** Modulation in the spinal cord refers to the process by which pain signals are altered, amplified, or inhibited before being transmitted to higher levels of the central nervous system. It involves interactions between different types of neurons, neurotransmitters, and neuromodulators within the spinal cord. Modulation plays a crucial role in shaping the transmission of pain signals and ultimately influencing pain perception.

The Gate Control Theory of pain modulation, proposed by Melzack and Wall in 1965, provides insight into how the brain manages and regulates pain signals. It also explains that the spinal cord functions as a "gate," capable of either facilitating or inhibiting the transmission of pain signals to the brain. The opening and closing of this gate depend on the interplay between large-diameter nerve fibres responsible for carrying pain signals.

- **Ascending Pathway** (transmission to the brain): From the spinal cord, the pain signals ascend through specific pathways towards higher brain centres for further processing and perception. The two major ascending pathways involved in pain transmission are the spinothalamic tract and the dorsal column-medial lemniscus pathway. The spinothalamic tract carries pain and temperature information. It consists of two main divisions: the lateral spinothalamic tract, which transmits fast pain and temperature signals, and the anterior spinothalamic tract, which carries slow pain and diffuse touch information. The Dorsal Column-Medial Lemniscus Pathway primarily carries sensory information about touch, vibration, and proprioception. However, it also plays a role in transmitting information about non-noxious temperatures and some aspects of pain.

- **Perception:** The modulated pain signals continue their journey from the spinal cord to the brainstem and then to the thalamus, which acts as a central relay station for sensory information. The thalamus acts as a relay station for sensory information, including pain signals, and directs these signals to various regions of the cerebral cortex for further processing.[3] The thalamus also filters and prioritises sensory information, allowing the brain to focus on pain signals that require immediate attention. Having received incoming pain signals from the spinal cord and other sensory pathways, it then relays them to specific cerebral cortex areas responsible for pain perception.

The cerebral cortex is the outer layer of the brain and is involved in higher-order cognitive functions, including the perception and interpretation of pain.[4] Different regions of the cerebral cortex are responsible for different aspects of pain perception. For example, the somatosensory cortex processes the location and intensity of pain, while the anterior cingulate cortex and insula are involved in the emotional and affective aspects of pain. The cerebral cortex, which is the brain's outermost layer, integrates pain signals with other sensory information, such as touch, temperature, and proprioception, allowing for a comprehensive *perception* of pain. It also engages in cognitive evaluation, drawing on past experiences and beliefs to interpret and assign meaning to the pain experience. Additionally, the cerebral cortex plays a role in the modulation of pain perception through descending pathways, which can influence the intensity and interpretation of pain signals.

The somatosensory cortex is within the cortex, where pain signals are transmitted. The somatosensory cortex is responsible for processing and interpreting sensory information related to touch, temperature, pain, and proprioception. With pain, the somatosensory cortex allows the person to perceive and localise the pain intensity and quality.

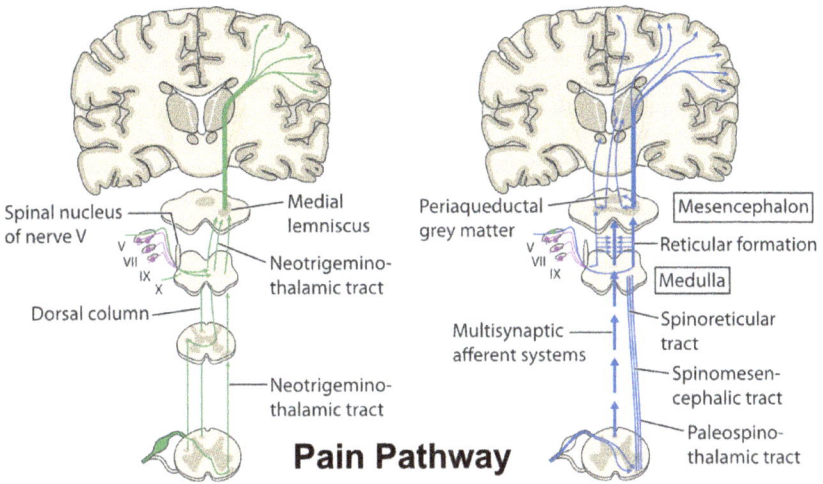

Spinal nucleus of nerve V — Medial lemniscus

Neotrigemino-thalamic tract

Dorsal column

Neotrigemino-thalamic tract

V VII IX X

Periaqueductal grey matter — Mesencephalon

Reticular formation

Medulla

V VII IX

Multisynaptic afferent systems

Spinoreticular tract

Spinomesen-cephalic tract

Paleospino-thalamic tract

Pain Pathway

Measuring Pain

As pain, which is an important symptom, is subjective, there is no scientific way to measure pain. Nevertheless, devices such as a dolorimeter have been used to measure sensitivity to pain and tolerance to pain. The device applies stimulus such as pressure, heat or electric current to produce a sensation (pain) which is then measured. A dolorimeter is not frequently used as it is not considered a reliable source of pain measurement. The standard method of recording pain used are;

i) Numerical rating scale from 0 to 10, where 0 is no pain, and 10 is the worst pain.

ii) Faces scale using several pictures showing different moods of pain.

iii) McGill Pain Questionnaire, which uses groups of words to describe pain.

MEDICAL PAIN SCALE

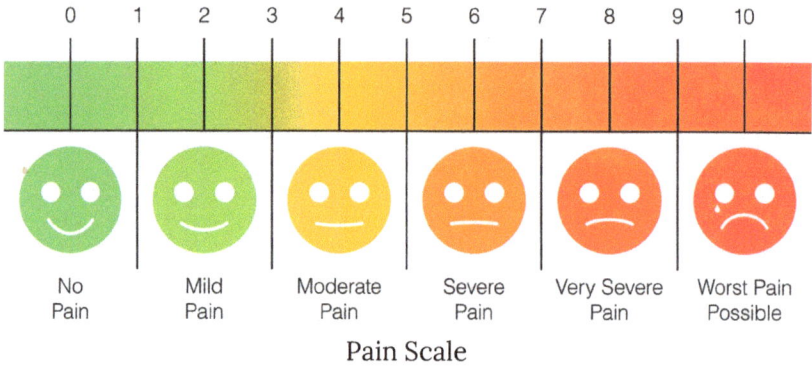

| 0 | 1 | 2 | 3 | 4 | 5 | 6 | 7 | 8 | 9 | 10 |

| No Pain | Mild Pain | Moderate Pain | Severe Pain | Very Severe Pain | Worst Pain Possible |

Pain Scale

A Note on Nonsteroidal Anti-Inflammatory Drugs (NSAIDs)

Nonsteroidal Anti-inflammatory drugs (NSAIDs) are a class of medications which are commonly used to alleviate pain, reduce inflammation, and also lower fever. Unlike steroidal medications, NSAIDs work by inhibiting enzymes known as cyclooxygenases (COX enzymes). These enzymes play a role in the production of chemicals called prostaglandins, which are involved in processes like pain perception, inflammation, and fever.

NSAIDs are popular among athletes as they quickly reduce pain and inflammation. This is mainly seen with professional athletes who are often under pressure to return to sports early despite their injury not being fully healed. Studies have shown that professional athletes are 3.6 times more likely to use NSAIDs than the general population.[5]

How NSAIDs work

As seen previously, inflammation is the body's natural reaction to injury or harmful stimuli, and prostaglandins are central to this process. When tissues are injured, a type of fatty acid called arachidonic acid is released from cell membranes. The arachidonic acid is then transformed into prostaglandin H2 by enzymes called cyclooxygenases (COX enzymes). Prostaglandins have various effects that contribute to the inflammatory response. They encourage vasodilation, which increases blood flow to the affected area, causing redness and warmth. Prostaglandins also increase the permeability of blood vessel walls, enabling immune cells, antibodies, and nutrients to enter tissues, resulting in swelling or oedema, all related to inflammation.

NSAIDs, exert their effect on the inflammatory process by targeting the COX enzymes (responsible for producing prostaglandins). By inhibiting the activity of these enzymes, NSAIDs effectively reduce the production of prostaglandins.[6] This reduction leads to a decrease in key inflammatory effects, including pain, swelling, redness, and fever.

Additionally, NSAID's act as potent pain relievers by mitigating the sensitization of nerve endings by prostaglandins. They do this by alleviating the intensity of pain signals, offering relief from discomfort. NSAIDs can also help lower fever by reducing the production of fever-inducing prostaglandins in the brain's hypothalamus.

Apart from their role in inflammation, prostaglandins also act as mediators for various physiologic functions protecting the stomach lining and regulating blood pressure. The negative effect of inhibiting prostaglandins may range from dyspepsia to upper gastrointestinal bleeds and potential cardiovascular side effects, including myocardial infarction.

Recently, particularly amongst keen amateurs and elite endurance athletes, there has been a worrying trend of using ibuprofen and other NSAIDs to reduce muscle pain both before an endurance event such as a marathon and after exercise to aid recovery of muscles so that they can compete with the highest intensity and for a longer duration. Studies have shown that using NSAIDs in this manner is of insignificant benefit and is associated with exertional hyponatremia (reduced sodium in the blood), which is related to altered renal function and reduced fluid transport leading to dehydration and also kidney failure.

Conclusion

Understanding Western Medicine's pain mechanisms is important for TCM practitioner as it enables a more comprehensive assessment of a patient's condition, ensuring safety and identifying when Western Medical intervention may be necessary. This knowledge allows for the integration of TCM and Western modalities for more effective pain management. Additionally, it facilitates clear communication with Western healthcare providers and offers patients with informed decision-making. Overall, the understanding of Western Medicine mechanism of pain enables TCM practitioners to offer well-rounded, safe, and effective pain management.

References

1. www:physio-pedia.com/Chronic_Disease
2. www:practicalpainmanagement.com/conceptual-model-pain
3. Yaksh TL. Pharmacology of spinal adrenergic systems which modulate spinal nociceptive processing. *Pharmacology Biochemistry and Behavior.* 1985
4. www:courses.lumenlearning.com/waymaker-psychology/chapter/reading-parts-of-the-brain
5. Alaranta A, Alaranta H, Heliövaara M, Airaksinen M, Helenius I. Ample use of physician-prescribed medications in Finnish elite athletes. Int J Sports Med. 2006;27(11):919–25
6. www:ncbi.nlm.nih.gov/pmc/articles/PMC6039135.

Chapter 5

Pain: Traditional Chinese Medicine Perspective

In Traditional Chinese Medicine, Qi is a fundamental concept representing vital energy that flows through the body and the universe. It is both a tangible substance and a dynamic force that sustains life and drives physiological functions. TCM recognises various types of Qi, such as Yuan Qi (Original Qi), Zong Qi (derived from air and food), Ying Qi (Nutritive Qi), and Wei Qi (Defensive Qi). Optimal health is achieved when Qi flows harmoniously, while imbalances can lead to health issues.

In Traditional Chinese Medicine the understanding of pain extends beyond mere physical discomfort. It is a manifestation of underlying imbalances in the body's vital energies, meridians and organ systems. TCM recognizes a diverse range of conditions that can give rise to pain, each associated with specific patterns of disharmony. These patterns encompass disruptions in the flow of Qi and Blood, as well as imbalances in Yin and Yang and Bi Syndrome.

Blood, in TCM, is responsible for nourishing and moisturising the organs and tissues, supporting mental functions, building and maintaining bodily structures, and ensuring proper circulation of nutrients and oxygen. Additionally, Blood supports menstruation and reproduction in women and harmonises emotions and the mind. When Blood flow is impaired, such as in Blood Stasis, pain is experienced.

Qi and Blood are closely connected and interdependent substances, each playing crucial roles in the body's functioning. Qi represents the vital energy and Blood encompasses not only the physical Blood but also nourishing fluids that support the body's structure and provide essential nutrients. The relationship between Qi and Blood in TCM involves mutual influence so that Qi propels the movement of Blood, ensuring proper circulation. Blood nourishes Qi, providing the material basis for its generation and maintenance.

The terms Blood Stasis and Blood Stagnation referred to below are used interchangeably to describe a condition where the circulation of blood becomes obstructed or sluggish, leading to the accumulation of Stagnant Blood in certain areas of the body. Both terms are to convey the idea that Blood is not flowing smoothly as it should.

1) Qi Stagnation and Pain

Qi Stagnation can result from injury, overuse, or emotional stress. This stagnation causes blockages along the meridians and affected tissues. As a consequence of this, the smooth flow of Qi is hindered, causing pain and discomfort. The pain is typically characterised as dull and persistent, concentrated in specific areas. Additionally, Qi stagnation may induce muscle spasms and tension, intensifying the pain and causing tightness and reduced flexibility in the affected muscles.

Symptoms of Qi Stagnation:

- Qi Stagnation is often associated with emotional symptoms such as irritability, mood swings, anxiety, and a tendency to feel frustrated or stuck.

- Stagnant Qi can lead to physical discomfort, such as a sensation of fullness or distension in the chest, abdomen or a feeling of tightness. The patient may also have a sensation of a "lump in the throat"

- Stagnation of Qi is linked to pain, particularly dull and achy pain that moves or changes in intensity. In females, it might also manifest as menstrual cramps, tension headaches, or pain in the ribcage or flank area. In females, Qi stagnation can sometimes manifest as breast tenderness or distension, particularly in the premenstrual phase.

- For females, Qi stagnation contributes to menstrual irregularities, including changes in flow, mood swings, and abdominal discomfort during menstruation.

- Qi Stagnation can affect digestion, leading to symptoms such as bloating, belching, abdominal discomfort, and irregular bowel movements.

- Stagnant Qi can cause a feeling of fatigue or lethargy, as the smooth flow of energy throughout the body is disrupted.

- Difficulty falling asleep or staying asleep can be attributed to Qi stagnation, due to emotional unrest.

- Qi Stagnation can be linked to symptoms such as acid reflux, indigestion, and irregular appetite.

- Tension-type headaches that involve tightness or pressure around the head and neck can be related to Qi stagnation.

- Stagnant Qi can impact emotional well-being and also contributes to feelings of low moods and depression.

Qi Stagnation and Musculoskeletal and Sports Injuries

Qi Stagnation in musculoskeletal and sports injuries is characterized by a range of symptoms. These include pain, which is often described as dull, stabbing, or distending. Stiffness and limited range of motion are also common, particularly after periods of inactivity. Emotional stress can exacerbate these symptoms, leading to feelings of tightness and tension in the affected area. Patients may also experience palpable knots or nodules, and irregular sensations like fullness or pressure. Emotional manifestations such as irritability and mood swings are associated with Qi stagnation, along with potential digestive discomfort. Prolonged inactivity tends to worsen symptoms, making movement and exercise important for alleviating blockages and promoting Qi flow.

2) Blood Stasis and Pain

Following an injury or trauma, there is localised pooling or stagnation of Blood. This is usually a response to trauma or inflammation. Blood Stasis leads to pain that is sharp, stabbing, and intense. The pain may be aggravated by movement or pressure on the affected area. Stagnant Blood can cause the injured tissues to become congested and inflamed, further exacerbating the pain and delaying healing.

Symptoms of Blood Stasis:

- Blood Stasis often leads to localized or fixed pain that is sharp, stabbing, or severe in nature. The pain may be chronic.

- Areas of the skin affected by Blood Stasis might appear dark purple or bluish in colour. This discoloration is the result of poor Blood circulation.

- Blood Stasis can cause a feeling of coldness in the affected area due to reduced circulation.

- The development of varicose veins, which are twisted and enlarged veins, can be attributed to Blood Stasis.

- Blood Stasis can cause localized swelling or oedema due to the accumulation of fluids and impaired Blood flow.

- Patients with Blood Stasis might bruise easily and the bruises may take longer to heal.

- Blood Stasis is often associated with gynaecological issues, such as heavy or painful menstrual periods, clots in menstrual blood, or irregular cycles.

- Blood Stasis in the abdominal area can lead to feelings of bloating, distension, and discomfort.

- Reduced Blood flow caused by Blood Stasis can result in numbness or tingling in the affected area.

- Blood Stasis can impair the body's ability to heal wounds and injuries promptly.

- Blood Stasis can contribute to the formation of palpable masses or lumps in the body, which may be accompanied by pain.

Blood Stagnation and Musculoskeletal and Sports Injuries

Blood Stagnation in the context of musculoskeletal and sports injuries is characterized by specific symptoms. These include intense and sharp pain, which is often localized and exacerbated by movement. Visible signs may include bruising and hematomas, as well as a dark or purplish discoloration of the skin due to accumulated blood. The affected area may feel cold and may exhibit numbness or tingling sensations. Stiffness and reduced range of motion are common due to impaired circulation, and pain can worsen with pressure or palpation. Unlike Qi Stagnation, Blood Stagnation typically leads to fixed and localized pain patterns. Additionally, delayed healing of injuries may occur, and in advanced cases, palpable masses or nodules may be present.

Qi and Blood Stagnation

As explained above, Qi and Blood are closely connected and interdependent substances, each playing crucial roles in the body's functioning. Qi represents the vital energy that flows throughout the body, driving all physiological processes. On the other hand, Blood encompasses not only the physical blood but also nourishing fluids that support the body's structure providing essential nutrients. The relationship between Qi and Blood in TCM involves mutual influence so that Qi propels the movement of Blood, ensuring proper circulation. Blood nourishes Qi, providing the material basis for its generation and maintenance. Due to the interdependence between Qi and Blood, when Qi flow is interrupted, Blood flow is also interrupted, causing the common syndrome of Qi and Blood Stagnation, which causes pain. Qi and Blood stagnation can manifest in various symptoms and signs, depending on the areas and meridians affected.

When there is Qi and Blood Stagnation, often the symptoms will show varying degrees of the above symptoms.

3) QI and Blood Deficiency Pain

In TCM, a deficiency of Qi and Blood can contribute to the development of pain, as Qi and Blood are essential for nourishing muscles, tendons, and joints. When Qi is deficient, the tissues may not receive the necessary "energy" and support they require. Similarly, a deficiency of Blood means there is inadequate nourishment for the tissues. Without proper nourishment, the muscles and joints can become weakened and more prone to pain. When there is a lack or insufficiency of Qi and Blood, the body's ability to properly nourish and support the tissues is compromised, leading to pain and discomfort.

Qi and Blood are responsible for promoting healthy circulation throughout the body. When there is a deficiency, the circulation may become compromised. Insufficient Qi can result in sluggish movement of Blood, while Blood deficiency can cause a lack of volume or flow. Impaired circulation can lead to Qi and Blood Stagnation, manifesting as pain and discomfort in the muscles and joints, as discussed above.

When Qi and Blood are deficient, muscles and joints may lack support and stability, making them more susceptible to pain, strain, and injury.

Symptoms of Qi Deficiency:

- Persistent and unexplained fatigue or lack of energy is the classic symptom of Qi deficiency.

- Qi deficiency can lead to shortness of breath even with minimal physical exertion.

- Generalized weakness, especially in the muscles, is a common symptom of Qi deficiency.

- Qi deficiency might cause a pale or sallow complexion due to reduced blood flow.

- A decreased or irregular appetite can be attributed to Qi deficiency.

- The voice might become weak or easily fatigued in individuals with Qi deficiency.

- A weakened immune system and frequent illnesses can be related to Qi deficiency.

- Qi deficiency can lead to digestive symptoms such as bloating, gas, and loose stools.

- Reduced physical and mental stamina are common signs of Qi deficiency.

- Spontaneous sweating without engaging in physical activity or being in a warm environment might indicate Qi deficiency.

Symptoms of Blood Deficiency:

- Blood deficiency can result in a pale or washed-out complexion.

- Blood deficiency might cause dizziness, particularly upon standing up quickly.

- Chronic fatigue is a common symptom of blood deficiency.

- Weak and brittle nails and hair can be indicative of blood deficiency.

- Blood deficiency can lead to dry and flaky skin.

- Difficulty falling asleep or staying asleep can be related to blood deficiency.

- Females with blood deficiency might experience irregular or scanty menstrual periods.

- Heart palpitations or a sensation of irregular heartbeats might be associated with blood deficiency.

- Reduced blood flow due to blood deficiency can cause numbness or tingling sensations.

- Blood deficiency can lead to blurry vision or dry eyes.

Differences Between Stagnant and Deficient States

In Traditional Chinese Medicine, understanding the distinctions between Qi and Blood stagnation, as well as Qi and Blood deficiency, is essential in diagnosing and treating health conditions. Qi stagnation involves an obstruction in the flow of vital energy, resulting in symptoms like pain and emotional stress. Blood stagnation, conversely, pertains to a slowdown or blockage in the circulation of blood, leading to severe pain, visible bruising, and dark discoloration. Qi deficiency signifies a weakness in the body's vital energy, causing fatigue and weakness, while Blood deficiency denotes an insufficient blood supply, resulting in symptoms like pale skin and dizziness. Treatment approaches vary, aiming to restore balance, for example, Qi stagnation is addressed by promoting Qi flow, while Blood stagnation is treated by improving blood circulation. Qi and Blood deficiencies are managed by strengthening vital energy and nourishing the blood supply, respectively.

It is important to note that these conditions can overlap.

4) Pathogenic Factors as a Cause of Pain

External Pathogenic Factors are considered one of the causes of pain. TCM attributes pain to specific pathogenic external factors, such as Wind, Cold, Dampness, Heat, and Dryness, which can invade the body and disrupt its balance.

- Wind is considered one of the primary external pathogens that causes pain. Wind is characterised by its ability to move and change rapidly. In TCM theory, Wind can invade the body and cause pain by obstructing the smooth flow of Qi and Blood. Wind can also carry other pathogens, such as Cold or Dampness, which further contribute to pain. Wind invasion often results in sudden onset of pain that can move from one area to another.

- Cold is another common external pathogen that can cause pain. Cold has a constricting and contracting nature, which can hinder the flow of Qi and Blood, leading to pain and stiffness. Exposure to cold environments, drafts, or ingesting cold foods and beverages can contribute to the accumulation of Cold in the body, resulting in musculoskeletal pain.

- Dampness is characterised by its heavy, stagnant, and obstructive nature. It can arise from environmental factors like high humidity or living in damp conditions, as well as internal factors such as a weak digestive system (Spleen). Dampness can obstruct the flow of Qi and impede circulation, leading to pain and heaviness in the muscles and joints. Dampness can be challenging to treat.

- Heat refers to excessive heat or inflammation in the body. Heat arises from external exposure to factors such as hot environments or excessive sun exposure, as well as internal factors such as emotional stress or an imbalance in the body's internal systems. Heat can cause pain by generating inflammation and swelling in the affected area, leading to redness, heat sensations, and discomfort.

- Dryness is characterised by a lack of moisture and lubrication in the body. Dryness can be caused by external factors such as dry climates, excessive exposure to air conditioning or heating systems, and internal factors such as a deficiency of Yin fluids. Dryness can cause muscle and joint dryness, leading to pain and stiffness.

When the above External Pathogenic Factors invade the body, they disrupt the flow of Qi and Blood, obstruct the meridians, and cause pain and discomfort in the affected areas. TCM treatment aims to expel or resolve these pathogens from the body, restore the flow of Qi and Blood, and alleviate pain.

5) Meridian Imbalance Pain

In TCM, organ imbalances can lead to meridian or channel blockages as organs and meridians are closely interconnected. Meridians are pathways through which Qi and Blood flow to nourish organs and tissues. When an organ is imbalanced, it can cause stagnation or blockage in its corresponding meridian, disrupting the smooth flow of Qi and Blood. This can result in pain and discomfort. Factors such as Qi stagnation, Blood Stasis, Heat or Cold accumulation, Dampness or Phlegm and emotional factors can contribute to meridian blockages.

Pain symptoms associated with specific meridian imbalances:

- Liver meridian imbalance symptoms: Rib-side or flank pain, especially on the right side. The pain may feel dull and persistent, aggravated by emotional stress, anger, or frustration. There may also be accompanying symptoms such as mood swings, irritability, and headaches.

- Gallbladder meridian imbalance symptoms: Sharp or stabbing pain along the sides of the head (temples), the outer edges of the eyes, or the shoulders. The pain may be worsened by stress, indecision, or exposure to wind and drafts. It can be associated with symptoms like dizziness, blurred vision, and a bitter taste in the mouth.

- Heart meridian imbalance symptoms: Chest pain or discomfort, often described as a dull ache or pressure. The pain may radiate to the left arm and may be triggered or exacerbated by emotional turmoil, anxiety, or excessive joy. Palpitations, shortness of breath, and insomnia may accompany the pain.

- Lung meridian imbalance symptoms: Pain in the chest or shoulders, often accompanied by shortness of breath, coughing, or phlegm production. The pain may be aggravated by exposure to cold or windy weather and may be associated with respiratory issues such as asthma or bronchitis.

- Spleen meridian imbalance symptoms: Abdominal pain, bloating, and a sense of fullness in the epigastric region (upper abdomen). The pain may be worsened by consuming greasy or sweet foods, and there may be symptoms of poor digestion, fatigue, and loose stools.

- Stomach meridian imbalance symptoms: Epigastric pain or discomfort in midabdominal, worsened by stress, irregular eating habits, or overeating. There may be symptoms of acid reflux, belching, and nausea.

- Kidney meridian imbalance symptoms: Low back pain, knee weakness, and frequent urination. The pain may be worse during times of fatigue or overexertion. Additionally, there may be symptoms related to the urinary system, such as nocturia or difficulty urinating.

- Bladder meridian imbalance symptoms: Low back pain, pain, or discomfort along the back of the legs. The pain may be aggravated by prolonged sitting or standing, and there may be urinary issues, such as frequent or painful urination.

- Pericardium meridian imbalance symptoms: Chest pain or tightness, similar to heart meridian imbalance. The pain may be associated with emotional distress, anxiety, or emotional fluctuations. There may also be symptoms of palpitations and poor sleep.

- Triple Burner meridian imbalance symptoms: Pain and discomfort in the three sections of the body (upper, middle, and lower Jiao), affecting various organs and systems. Triple Burner imbalances may manifest as a generalised feeling of discomfort or pain without a clear local origin.

6) Yin and Yang Imbalance Pain

An imbalance between Yin and Yang energies can contribute to the development of pain. When there is an imbalance between Yin and Yang, the harmonious functioning of the body is disrupted, resulting in pain.

- Yin Deficiency: As Yin represents the nourishing, cooling, and moistening aspects of the body, when there is a deficiency of Yin, it means there is insufficient Yin energy to balance the Yang energy. Yin deficiency can be caused by chronic stress, overwork, excessive consumption of heated foods or beverages, or ageing. Yin deficiency can lead to heat or dryness in the body. This heat and dryness can cause inflammation, irritate the tissues, and result in pain and discomfort. Symptoms of Empty Heat may also be apparent.

- Yang Excess – As Yang represents the active, warming, and energising aspects of the body, when there is an excess of Yang, it means there is an imbalance towards excessive Yang energy. This can be caused by excessive physical activity, emotional agitation, or consuming too many warming foods or beverages. Excessive Yang can generate heat and inflammation, leading to pain. It can also cause excessive energy or tension in the muscles and joints, resulting in pain and stiffness.

Yin and Yang imbalances can also manifest as excessive Cold or constriction. Yin deficiency can lead to inadequate nourishing fluids, resulting in dryness and inflammation. Yang deficiency can cause a lack of warmth and vitality, leading to coldness and constriction in the muscles and joints. Coldness and constriction can restrict the flow of Qi and Blood, resulting in pain and stiffness.

Yin and Yang imbalances can disrupt the smooth flow of Qi in the body. An imbalance between Yin and Yang can obstruct Qi's flow, leading to pain and discomfort as Qi is responsible for maintaining the healthy functioning of the body's systems, including the muscles and joints.

7) Emotional Factors of Pain

In TCM, emotional factors such as stress, frustration, anger, sadness, or other intense emotions can disrupt Qi's smooth flow, causing it to become stagnant. When Qi becomes stagnant or blocked due to emotional factors, it can manifest as physical pain. Emotional imbalances can also cause increased muscle tension and "constrictions" in the body. For example, chronic stress or anxiety can lead to tense muscles, especially in the neck, shoulders, and back. Prolonged muscle tension can result in pain, stiffness, and reduced flexibility.

Emotion imbalance can also cause pain, as each emotion is associated with. specific organ systems in the body. For

TCM Pattern	Description of Sensation
Qi Stagnation	Distending or stabbing pain, often moving and aggravated by stress or emotions.
Blood Stasis	Sharp, stabbing pain that is fixed in location, often accompanied by dark or purple skin discoloration.
Qi and Blood Deficiency	Dull, achy pain that is diffuse and feels weak, worsened by fatigue or exertion.
Cold Invasion	Severe, sharp pain that is relieved by warmth, aversion to cold, stiffness.
Dampness and Phlegm	Dull, heavy pain with a sensation of fullness and swelling, worsened by damp weather.
Wind Invasion	Moving or migrating pain that changes location frequently, sensitivity to drafts.
Heat and Fire	Burning or throbbing pain with inflammation and redness, heat sensation.
Yang Deficiency	Dull, achy pain with a sensation of coldness, relief from warmth, low energy.
Yin Deficiency	Dull, nagging pain with a sensation of heat or burning, dryness, restlessness.

Table to Show TCM Pain Patterns.

instance, anger is related to the liver, sadness to the lungs, worry to the spleen, fear to the kidneys, and joy to the heart. When emotions are experienced in an extreme or prolonged manner, they can affect the corresponding organ systems, disrupting their functions and leading to pain or discomfort. The liver is susceptible to emotional stress and frustration in TCM. When emotions such as anger, irritability, or resentment are not effectively processed, they can cause stagnation of Liver Qi. Liver Qi Stagnation can manifest as pain, especially in the muscles, tendons, and joints. It can also contribute to conditions like tension headaches.

Traditional Chinese Medicine and Western Medicine Pain Differences

The explanation of pain in TCM differs from that of Western Medicine above in several key aspects:

- **TCM** takes a holistic approach to pain, considering the body, mind, and environment as an integrated whole. TCM views pain as a manifestation of underlying imbalances in the body's energy systems of Qi and Blood flow, meridian blockages, and Yin-Yang imbalances. Also, TCM considers various factors, such as emotions, lifestyle, and environmental influences, in understanding the causes and treatment of pain.

- **TCM** recognises that each person is unique, with their constitution, patterns of disharmony, and specific symptoms, so tailoring diagnosis and treatment to the individual, taking into account the person's overall health, constitution, and specific manifestations of pain. Therefore, TCM treatment is personalised and may involve a combination of therapies, including acupuncture, herbal medicine, dietary recommendations, and lifestyle modifications.

- **TCM** identifies a network of meridians through which Qi and Blood flow. Pain in TCM is explained by blockages and disruptions in the meridians. Acupuncture points are used in TCM to stimulate specific points along the meridians to regulate Qi flow and Blood to alleviate pain. Therefore, TCM treatments aim to restore Qi's balance and smooth flow to alleviate pain.

- In contrast, Western Medicine primarily focuses on the physical and physiological aspects of pain. It often explains pain based on anatomical structures, physiological processes, and pathological conditions. Western Medicine typically utilises diagnostic tools, imaging techniques, and laboratory tests to identify the underlying causes of pain, such as tissue damage, inflammation, or nerve dysfunction. Treatment approaches in Western Medicine include medication, surgery, physical therapy, and interventions targeted at the physiological mechanisms involved in pain.

While Western Medicine and TCM have different approaches and perspectives on pain, they should not be mutually exclusive. By integrating both approaches, taking advantage of and strengths of each system to provide comprehensive care and address pain from multiple angles. For the TCM practitioner, this involves having an understanding of Western Medicine.

TCM and Pain Control - Various Hypothesis

Various models and concepts have been postulated, which are thought to explain how TCM may control and relieve pain.

- **Local Blood Flow.**

  When acupuncture needles are inserted into an area of the body, the trauma created causes an inflammatory response, increasing blood flow to the area and promoting healing by providing nourishment.[1] The chemicals cause vasodilation and improve vascular permeability. The cumulative effect of this is to encourage the removal of inflammatory chemicals but enhance healing mediators in the area.[2]

It is also thought that the effect of needling, as the acupuncture needle is a "foreign" object, this action may act to elevate adrenocorticotrophic hormone, which suggests adrenal activation and the release of endogenous corticosteroids, which directly reduce pain.

- **Trigger Point or Dry Needling.**

Trigger point therapy is a neuromuscular therapy which is used to control pain. Using dry needling, an acupuncture needle is inserted into a sensitive area or knot in the muscle to desensitise the muscle or the knot. There is an opinion that trigger points may have similarities to Ah Shi (also referred to as Ashi) points, frequently used in acupuncture.

- **Neuro-gate Pain Theory.**

It is believed that when inserting acupuncture needles, this may affect the peripheral nervous system by blocking the conduction of impulses in the sensory fibres and also inhibiting the downward conduction from the dorsal horn cell of the spinal cord (Lu Guowe 1979 and Qiu Maoling 1989). The effect of this is to inhibit or block pain. The nerve fibres likely to be affected are types II, III, and IV.

Type II are cutaneous mechano-receptors and nociceptors.

Type III are free nerve endings of touch, pressure, and cold.

Type IV are the nociceptors (multi-receptive nociceptors).

- **Endorphins and Opioids.**

When acupuncture needles are inserted, the minor trauma causes the release of pain-relieving chemicals at the insertion site, spinal cord, and brain. Endorphins and opioids are thought to be released, which have the effect of reducing or blocking the levels of pain perceived.[3]

- **Electro acupuncture**

Serotonin is a neurotransmitter which has the effect of influencing pain sensitivity. In a study (Zhu Dinger), higher serotonin levels were detected in the thalamus, medulla oblongata and midbrain when electroacupuncture was used. Serotonin had the effect of sedating pain.

Several other hypotheses have demonstrated the efficacy of acupuncture in sedating and relieving pain. Unfortunately, no substantial clinical trials have been carried out to demonstrate the mechanism of how acupuncture works for pain relief. However, with increasing patient satisfaction and increased referrals from Western Medicine doctors for acupuncture, there can be little doubt that using acupuncture to alleviate or moderate pain can help the athlete recover from injuries.

TCM Objectives of Pain Control

- Either complete relief from pain or reduce the level of pain experienced.
- Increase in mobility.
- Enhancing quality of life, especially for chronic and idiopathic pain.
- Alleviate accompanying pain symptoms such as anger, anxiety, and stress.
- Reduce reliance and dependency on painkillers. This objective must always be considered in collaboration with the patient's medical practitioner (if on prescribed medication).

Conclusion

Unlike Western Medicine, TCM offers a simple explanation of the factors causing pain. Concepts such as Qi, Blood, Yin and Yang are simple to understand and yet provide a mechanism for understanding pain, which can be treated effectively.

As a natural therapy, TCM treatment for pain (and inflammation) has several advantages compared to using drug therapies. TCM has no unwanted side effects and is effective and economical. TCM considers injuries and pain holistically, appreciating that emotions and the patient's mental state can affect the athlete's performance. Think of emotions such as anger and anxiety, common amongst professional athletes as they participate in an ever-increasing competitive environment. These emotions can harm the Liver, affecting the free flow of Qi. When Liver Qi and Blood become deficient, tendons will not be nourished, limiting joint movement and making the area more prone to injury. Thus, when treating athletes for injuries, TCM takes a holistic approach rather than a regimental and generalised prescribed approach of Western Medicine.

References

1. Kapthuk T J. Acupuncture theory, efficacy, and practice. Ann Inter Med 2002; 136: 378-383.
2. Eur J App Physiol, 2003; 90(1-2): 114-119
3. Curr Opin Pharmacol. 2001; 1(1): 62-65

Chapter 6

Contrasting Philosophies of Traditional Chinese Medicine (TCM) & Western Medicine

TCM and Western Medicine Philosophies

When diagnosing and treating musculoskeletal and sports injuries, there are contrasting philosophical approaches in Traditional Chinese Medicine and Western Medicine. Sometimes, TCM practitioners may inadvertently blend Western Medicine perspectives with TCM principles, resulting in less effective outcomes for these conditions. *The key lies in understanding the fundamental differences between these two diverse medical systems, as their philosophies significantly differ.* By gaining a profound understanding of these distinctions, TCM treatment of musculoskeletal and sports injuries can be approached more insightfully and effectively. An understanding of these diverse approaches is crucial when dealing with musculoskeletal and sports injuries. By respecting the distinctiveness of each system and tailoring treatments accordingly, practitioners can optimise patient outcomes. Integrating the strengths of both TCM and Western Medicine can lead to more comprehensive and successful management of these injuries.

1. **Traditional Chinese Medicine** takes a holistic view, seeing the human body as a dynamic and interconnected system, where physical, emotional, mental, and spiritual aspects are interconnected and influence one another. Qi represents this interconnectedness, the vital energy that

flows through meridians, linking different organs and systems in the body. TCM regards the body as a microcosm of the universe, with the principles of Yin and Yang governing the balance and harmony of all living beings.

In Western Medicine, there is a reductionist perspective, where the human body is dissected into its components, including organs, tissues, cells, and molecules. This approach aims to comprehend diseases at the cellular and molecular levels, employing scientific research, clinical trials, and evidence-based methods for diagnosis and treatment. The primary focus lies in understanding the physical and biochemical mechanisms underlying diseases.

2. **In TCM**, individualised approach is a cornerstone of patient care. TCM recognises that each person is unique and complex, influenced by various internal external and environmental factors. These factors include one's constitution, genetic makeup, lifestyle choices, emotional state, environmental conditions, and past medical history. Therefore, TCM practitioners approach each patient as an individual with their own distinct pattern of health and disease.

    TCM practitioners assess the patient's symptoms, medical history, tongue appearance, pulse qualities, and other relevant signs during the diagnostic process. This comprehensive evaluation helps identify specific patterns of disharmony or imbalances within the body. TCM diagnosis involves identifying syndromes or patterns based on the principles of Yin and Yang, the Five Elements, and the flow of Qi and Blood. By understanding the underlying pattern of disharmony, TCM practitioners can determine the root cause of the illness. The focus shifts from simply addressing the outward symptoms to understanding the deeper imbalances contributing to the disease manifestation including the effects of the environment.

Once the diagnosis is established, a personalised treatment plan is formulated for the individual. TCM treatments encompass a variety of modalities, such as acupuncture, herbal medicine, dietary recommendations, lifestyle modifications, and mind-body practices like Tai Chi or Qi Gong.

By customising the treatment to the individual's specific needs, TCM aims to support the body's innate healing capacity and restore harmony. This individualised approach recognises that the same disease can manifest differently in different people due to their unique constitutions and life circumstances. By addressing the root cause of the illness and supporting the body's self-regulating mechanisms, TCM seeks to achieve long-term healing and prevent the recurrence of the disease.

In Western Medicine, a standardised approach is employed for diagnosing and treating various diseases. This approach involves using established diagnostic criteria and guidelines developed based on scientific research, clinical trials, and evidence-based practices. These standardised criteria and protocols serve as essential tools for healthcare professionals in their decision-making process when evaluating patients and determining the most appropriate course of treatment.

When a patient presents with symptoms, healthcare providers in Western Medicine follow a systematic process of gathering relevant medical history, conducting physical examinations, and ordering specific laboratory tests or imaging studies. The results of these diagnostic tests are then compared against established criteria to identify the presence of a particular disease or condition.

Once a diagnosis is confirmed, Western Medicine healthcare providers refer to standardised treatment protocols that outline the most effective and evidence-based interventions for managing the specific disease.

3. **Traditional Chinese Medicine** considers organs more than just physical structures; they are functional systems with unique properties and energetic functions. Each organ is associated with a specific meridian or channel through which Qi flows, connecting various body parts. Organs are seen as interrelated and interconnected, with their interactions playing a critical role in maintaining the body's overall health and balance. For example, the Liver is associated with the Liver meridian, and its functions extend beyond the anatomical Liver to regulate emotions and Qi's smooth flow throughout the body.

   In Western Medicine, organs are primarily understood from an anatomical and physiological perspective. The focus is on comprehending the structures and functions of organs as isolated entities without consideration of energetic flows or meridians. Western Medicine primarily studies the anatomical features, biochemical processes, and physiological functions of organs as they contribute to bodily processes.

4. **TCM** utilises specific and descriptive terminology to describe patterns of disharmony that underlie various health conditions. These terminologies are based on observations and interpretations of symptoms and signs associated with specific organ imbalances. For instance:

   Liver Qi Stagnation refers to a condition where the flow of Qi in the Liver meridian is blocked, leading to emotional symptoms like irritability and physical symptoms like abdominal distension. Kidney Yin Deficiency indicates a lack of Yin (nourishing and cooling aspect) in the Kidney system, which may manifest in symptoms such as hot flushes and night sweats. Dampness refers to an accumulation of stagnant and heavy fluids in the body, resulting in symptoms like oedema and a feeling of heaviness.

Western Medicine employs standardised diagnostic terminology based on specific diseases and conditions. Diagnoses are made according to established classification systems, which categorise illnesses based on their symptoms and objective findings. For example, Type 2 Diabetes Mellitus is a specific diagnosis of high blood sugar levels and insulin resistance.

5. **TCM** treatments focus on restoring the body's balance and harmony by regulating the flow of Qi and addressing the underlying patterns of disharmony, using acupuncture needles on specific points along the meridians to promote balanced Qi flow. Herbal medicine is prescribed to nourish or clear specific organ systems, and dietary adjustments and lifestyle modifications are recommended to support overall health. TCM treatments for muscular and sports injuries focus on restoring Qi and Blood flow, resolving stagnation and imbalances, and promoting the body's natural healing processes. To ensure overall balance and well-being, TCM treatments often consider the whole body's health, not just the injured area. Pain is seen as a symptom of underlying imbalances, and the goal is to treat the root cause of the pain rather than just masking the symptoms.

Western Medicine treatments for muscular and sports injuries are primarily targeted at managing the physical aspects of the injury. Physical therapies, such as physiotherapy and rehabilitative exercises, aim to strengthen and rehabilitate the injured muscles and tissues. Medications may be prescribed to manage pain and inflammation; in severe cases, surgical interventions may be necessary to repair damaged structures. Approach to pain management often relies on medications such as pain relievers and anti-inflammatories to manage pain. These medications target pain receptors and reduce inflammation, providing symptomatic relief. Physical therapies and modalities may also be used for pain management, but the emphasis is on addressing the physical source of pain.

6. **TCM** places a strong emphasis on preventive care and maintaining overall well-being. TCM preventive measures include lifestyle modifications, dietary recommendations, stress management, and mind–body practices like Tai Chi or Qi Gong. By fostering a balanced lifestyle and harmonious interactions with the environment, TCM aims to prevent the development of diseases and promote longevity.

   In Western Medicine preventive medicine is also essential, focusing on vaccinations, health screenings, and lifestyle modifications to reduce the risk of developing certain diseases. Preventive measures are often based on scientific evidence and public health strategies to enhance population health and well-being.

7. **In TCM** diagnosis, subjective data gathered through direct patient interaction plays a crucial role. Practitioners observe the patient's appearance, listen to their voice and speech patterns, palpate the pulse, and inspect the tongue to gain insights into the individual's health. Emotions, lifestyle, and overall constitution are also considered to comprehensively to understand the patient's condition.

   In Western Medicine, objective data that can be measured and quantified is given prominence. Diagnostic tools, such as laboratory tests, imaging studies (X-rays, MRI, CT scans), and vital signs (blood pressure, heart rate, temperature), are utilised to gather objective information about the patient's health. Evidence-based research guides Western medical diagnoses and treatment decisions.

Note on Syndrome Differentiation

Syndrome differentiation is a fundamental and essential aspect of TCM diagnosis and treatment. It refers to the process of identifying specific patterns of disharmony in the body based on a comprehensive analysis of a patient's signs, symptoms, medical history, and constitution.

The advantage of using syndrome differentiation is that the treatment approach is personalised, recognising the uniqueness of each individual and how diseases may present differently in different people. This allows the practitioner to tailor treatments based on the specific patterns of disharmony present in each patient, leading to better outcomes. Furthermore, as TCM places great emphasis on identifying and addressing the root cause of an illness rather than merely alleviating its symptoms, syndrome differentiation plays a vital role in pinpointing the underlying imbalances in the body's Qi, Blood, Yin, Yang, and other essential substances. By targeting the root cause, TCM treatments facilitate more sustainable and long-lasting patient health improvements. Another advantage of syndrome differentiation lies in its ability to guide TCM practitioners in selecting appropriate treatment modalities for each unique case. Based on the identified patterns of disharmony, practitioners can utilise acupuncture, herbal medicine, dietary adjustments, and lifestyle recommendations to address specific imbalances. This targeted approach enhances the therapeutic effect and reduces the risk of providing unnecessary or ineffective treatments, resulting in more precise and successful patient care.

In TCM, syndrome differentiation is crucial in diagnosing musculoskeletal and sports injuries. Apart from Qi, Blood, Yin, and Yang patterns, syndromes related to specific organs also apply in these cases. Injuries can also impact the smooth flow of Qi and Blood in the meridians associated with various organs, causing imbalances and affecting their functions, as described below;

Please note that organ injury or dysfunction referred to below in TCM is not structural damage but rather encompasses a wide range of imbalances, such as deficiency, excess, stagnation, or heat and cold patterns.

- The Liver is responsible for the smooth flow of Qi throughout the body. "Injuries" and emotional stress can lead to Liver Qi stagnation, causing muscle tension, irritability, and mood swings.

- The Spleen is involved in the transformation and transportation of Qi and Blood. "Injuries" can weaken the Spleen's function, leading to poor circulation, slow healing, and fatigue.

- The Kidneys govern the bones, joints, and connective tissues. "Injuries" can deplete Kidney Qi, resulting in weakness in the lower back and knees and susceptibility to musculoskeletal issues.

- The Heart governs the Blood and vessels. Severe "injuries" can lead to Blood Stasis, causing pain and swelling in the affected areas.

- The Lungs govern the skin and regulate the Wei Qi (defensive Qi). "Injuries" may affect the Lungs' ability to protect the body from external pathogens, making the person more susceptible to infections and Bi Syndromes.

- The Gallbladder meridian runs along the sides of the body and is susceptible to "injuries" in the hip and flank areas.

- The Stomach meridian runs down the front of the body and nourishes the muscles and tendons. "Injuries" can disrupt the flow of Qi and Blood in the Stomach meridian, leading to pain and weakness.

- The Bladder meridian runs along the back of the body and is often affected by "injuries" to the back and spine.

How Musculoskeletal and Sports Injuries affect Vital Body Substances

Qi and Blood Stagnation: In TCM, Qi represents the vital energy circulating throughout the body, while Blood nourishes the tissues and organs. A physical injury disrupts the smooth flow of both Qi and Blood in the affected region. This traumatic impact can lead to the stagnation of Qi, resulting in localised pain, tenderness, and swelling. Damage to blood vessels may cause the accumulation of Blood, leading to visible bruising and further stagnation. Such stagnation hampers the body's natural healing process, leading to prolonged pain and delayed recovery.

Meridian Flow: Meridians form intricate pathways through which Qi flows, connecting various organs and systems in the body. Physical injuries can create blockages or obstructions along these meridians, hindering the proper circulation of Qi. Consequently, the injured tissues may not receive adequate Qi and Blood supply, leading to slower healing and the development of chronic pain. Furthermore, the disruption in meridian flow can affect neighbouring meridians and organs, causing imbalances in the overall energy circulation throughout the body.

Yin and Yang Imbalance: Yin and Yang are fundamental concepts in TCM, representing the harmonious interplay of opposing forces in the body. Yang embodies warmth, activity, and movement, while Yin encompasses nourishment, rest, and cooling. Acute injuries often manifest with signs of Yang excess, such as heat, redness, and inflammation in the affected area. These symptoms signify the body's natural response to trauma, resulting in increased blood flow and warmth. However, if inflammation persists over an extended period, it can lead to a Yin deficiency, characterised by symptoms like dryness, weakness, and depleted energy.

Physical injuries impact the local area and can trigger systemic effects throughout the body. TCM recognises the interconnectedness of the body's systems, and a physical injury in one area may disrupt the flow of Qi and Blood in related meridians and organs. For instance, a knee injury may affect the Kidney and Liver meridians, causing imbalances in their respective functions and potentially giving rise to related symptoms in other body regions. This highlights the significance of considering the holistic impact of injuries on the entire body during the diagnostic and treatment processes in TCM.

In Traditional Chinese Medicine, understanding the impact of Musculoskeletal and Sports Injuries on vital body substances and organs helps differentiate syndromes and patterns. This understanding becomes the guiding principle in selecting appropriate acupuncture points for treatment. By assessing the disruptions in Qi, Blood, Yin, and Yang caused by injuries, TCM practitioners can determine the specific imbalances in the body. Based on this differentiation, the practitioner can then apply acupuncture to specific points along the meridians to restore balance, promote healing, and address the root cause of the injury effectively.

Acute, Subacute and Chronic Conditions

In both TCM and Western Medicine, the terms "acute," "subacute," and "chronic" refer to distinct stages of an illness or injury. However, the two medical systems' interpretations and approaches to these stages differ.

TCM Interpretation of Acute

In TCM, the acute stage is often termed the "excess" stage. It emerges with sudden symptom onset and stagnation of Qi,

Blood and an abundance of pathogenic factors, such as external pathogens, Wind, Cold, or Damp invading the body.

The acute stage is the early phase of a disease or injury, characterised by sudden symptoms. Acute conditions often develop rapidly and can be intense or severe. The duration of the acute stage varies depending on the specific condition but typically lasts for a few days. During this stage, the body's natural defence mechanisms actively respond to the illness or injury.

The primary objective of TCM treatment during this phase is to expel the pathogenic factors, resolve stagnation, and restore the normal flow of Qi and Blood.

TCM Interpretation of Subacute

The subacute stage follows the acute phase and is a transitional period between the acute and chronic stages. In TCM, the subacute stage is perceived as the "deficiency" stage. Symptoms may persist during this stage but are generally less severe than in the acute stage. Subacute conditions typically last for several weeks. At this point, the body's healing process is underway, and symptoms may gradually improve.

This stage focuses on replenishing and tonifying Qi, Blood, and Yin to strengthen the body's resistance and promote recovery.

TCM Interpretation of Chronic

The chronic stage is also considered a "deficiency" stage in TCM. It ensues when the body's vital energy and resources have been depleted over an extended period. Chronic conditions may result from unresolved acute or subacute issues or long-term imbalances in the body.

The chronic stage is the prolonged or long-term phase of a disease or injury. In chronic conditions, symptoms persist for an extended period, usually over three months, and may fluctuate in intensity. Chronic conditions often require ongoing management and may not have a definitive cure.

The treatment approach during the chronic stage is to tonify and nourish the deficient organs and vital substances, such as Qi, Blood, Yin, and Yang. TCM treatments aim to address the root cause of the chronic condition and restore the body's natural balance and harmony.

In Western Medicine

The terms "acute," "subacute," and "chronic" in Western Medicine refer to the duration and progression of an illness or injury.

Acute

In Western Medicine, the acute stage denotes the initial phase of an illness or injury, typically characterised by a sudden onset of symptoms. The focus during this stage is on diagnosing and treating the immediate cause of the illness or injury. Acute treatments often aim to control symptoms, reduce inflammation, and promote healing.

Subacute

The subacute stage in Western Medicine is an intermediate phase that follows the acute stage. During this period, symptoms may persist but are less severe than in the acute stage. Subacute treatments focus on managing symptoms, supporting healing, and preventing complications.

Chronic

The chronic stage in Western Medicine refers to the long-term phase of an illness or injury that lasts for an extended period. Chronic conditions may have developed from unresolved acute or subacute issues or may be caused by underlying health conditions. Treatment of chronic conditions aims to manage symptoms, improve quality of life, and address the condition's underlying causes to prevent further deterioration.

As TCM and Western Medicine recognise the different stages of an illness or injury, their treatment approaches and philosophies on addressing these stages can vary significantly. In the chapters that follow this chapter, please note that it is TCM's definition of "Acute", "Subacute", and "Chronic", which is used (for acupuncture point selection). So TCM treatment suggestions for each phase are based on TCM principles and do not necessarily correspond directly to Western Medicine conditions.

Examples of the Differences in Conditions seen in TCM and Western Medicine

- *Sprained Ankle*: A sprained ankle may be diagnosed as a Qi and Blood stagnation pattern in TCM. The injury leads to localised pain, swelling, and difficulty in weight-bearing. Treatment aims to promote the smooth flow of Qi and Blood to reduce pain and inflammation.

- *Tennis Elbow*: TCM diagnosis for tennis elbow might involve identifying an excess of Liver Qi and Wind-Heat invading the meridians. This can result in pain and inflammation around the elbow area. Treatment would focus on dispersing Wind-Heat and soothing Liver Qi to alleviate symptoms.

- *Muscle Strain*: A muscle strain could lead to a Qi and Blood stagnation pattern in TCM. Symptoms may include localised pain, tightness, and reduced flexibility. Treatment involves promoting circulation and relieving stagnation to aid in the healing process.

- *Knee Ligament Injury* (e.g., ACL Tear): In TCM, knee ligament injuries might be associated with a Kidney Qi and Blood deficiency pattern. This could lead to chronic instability and weakness in the knee joint. TCM treatment aims to tonify Kidney Qi and nourish Blood to support ligament healing.

- *Hamstring Strain*: A hamstring strain can lead to a pattern of Cold-Damp invasion in TCM. Symptoms may include pain and tightness in the back of the thigh, exacerbated by cold and damp weather. Treatment involves dispelling Cold-Dampness and promoting warmth and circulation in the affected area.

- *Carpal Tunnel Syndrome*: TCM diagnosis for carpal tunnel syndrome may involve identifying a pattern of Liver Qi stagnation and Phlegm obstruction. This can lead to wrist pain, numbness, and tingling in the fingers. Treatment aims to soothe Liver Qi, resolve Phlegm, and promote circulation to relieve symptoms.

- *Achilles Tendinitis*: Achilles tendinitis may be diagnosed as a pattern of Damp-Heat accumulation in the tendon. This can lead to pain, redness, and swelling in the back of the ankle. Treatment involves clearing Damp-Heat, reducing inflammation, and supporting tendon healing.

- *Muscle Contusion*: TCM diagnosis for a muscle contusion may involve identifying a pattern of Blood stasis and Qi stagnation. This can lead to localised pain, bruising, and swelling in the injured area. Treatment aims to promote Blood circulation, disperse stasis, and alleviate pain.

- *Plantar Fasciitis*: In TCM, plantar fasciitis might be associated with a pattern of Kidney Yin deficiency and Dampness accumulation. This can lead to heel pain, especially in the morning. Treatment focuses on nourishing Kidney Yin, resolving Dampness, and promoting healing.

Conclusion

Integrating Western Medicine using Western Medical diagnostics and TCM principles in treating musculoskeletal and sports injuries holds immense potential for optimising patient care and outcomes. By combining the strengths of both medical systems, TCM practitioners can offer a holistic and tailored approach that considers each individual's unique needs and characteristics.

Chapter 7

Trigger Point Therapy

Trigger points, also referred to as muscle knots or myofascial trigger points, are discrete, focal, hyperirritable spots located in a taut band of skeletal muscle or its surrounding fascia. These points have the potential to induce pain, discomfort, and even pain that is felt in other areas of the body when subjected to pressure or stimulation. Trigger points are thought to arise due to factors such as excessive use of the muscle, injury, or tension. When a muscle is repeatedly engaged, or if it remains in a contracted state for an extended period, it can lead to the formation of trigger points.

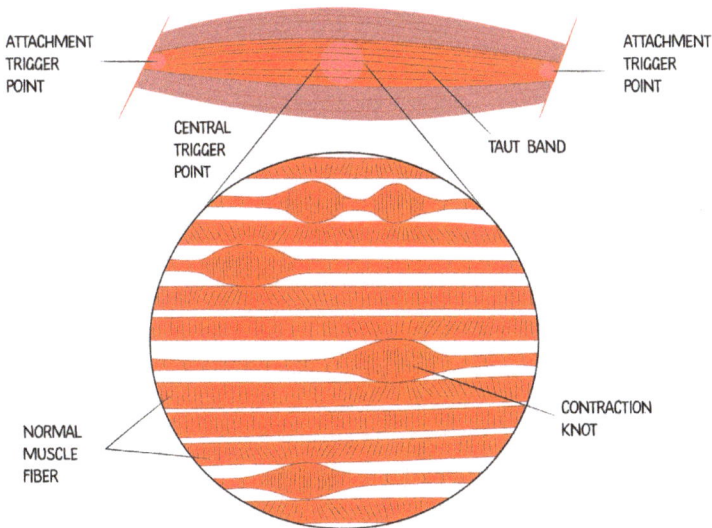

Trigger Points

Trigger point therapy and Dry needling are techniques used for musculoskeletal pain. The two techniques, although similar, have different therapeutic approaches. Trigger point therapy is a therapy used to alleviate musculoskeletal pain by identifying and treating trigger points. Trigger point therapy techniques include applying pressure, massage, stretching, and physical therapy. Dry needling, on the other hand, is a therapeutic technique which involves inserting fine acupuncture needles, into trigger points or tight muscle bands. The aim is to alleviate pain and enhance muscle function. This technique is "dry," meaning no substances are injected. Dry needling stimulates relaxation of muscle fibres, reducing pain and improving blood flow. It is also used for musculoskeletal issues.

In contrast trigger point injection (TPI) is a medical procedure employed for alleviating pain in specific muscle areas housing trigger points. In the process of a trigger point injection, a qualified and trained healthcare professional uses a small needle to administer a blend of local anaesthetic (such as lidocaine) and occasionally a corticosteroid (a medication with anti-inflammatory properties) directly into the trigger point. The objective of this injection is to mitigate pain and diminish inflammation within the affected muscle.

Trigger point therapy and dry needling have evolved over time, and they don't have single pioneer although Travell and Simons played a key role in developing trigger point therapy. However, the concept of trigger points can be traced back to the 19th century to Gowers, a physician and Sherrington a neurologist who made early observations regarding the relationship between muscular pain and specific points on the body. Since its early days, the therapy has gradually become integrated into mainstream medicine and is a major component of pain management. Dry needling, with similarities to acupuncture, developed in the 20th century in Western Medicine. Travell also contributed to early concepts of dry needling. Both therapies have been refined and expanded upon by numerous healthcare professionals over the years.

Types of Trigger Points

There are essentially two broad forms of Trigger Points, Active and Latent trigger points.

i) Active trigger points

Active trigger points can be classified into two main types; *primary trigger points* and *secondary trigger points.*

- *Primary trigger* points are specific areas in muscles and facia that have heightened sensitivity or tightness and directly cause pain and discomfort. Secondary trigger points develop in response to primary trigger points and are found in nearby or interconnected muscles. These secondary trigger points can contribute to the occurrence of *referred* pain and dysfunction in the affected area.

- *Secondary trigger* points arise in nearby or connected muscles as a compensatory reaction to the pain and dysfunction caused by the primary trigger points. They tend to form in muscles that work together or are functionally related to the muscles containing the primary trigger points. The development of secondary trigger points can create a cycle of referred pain and dysfunction, further contributing to the overall discomfort experienced by the individual. Treating primary and secondary trigger points is vital for managing myofascial pain effectively. When carrying out treatment, both primary and secondary trigger points should be treated for effective pain relief. Neglecting secondary trigger points may lead to incomplete pain management and a higher risk of recurrence. Therefore, a comprehensive pain assessment, including referred pain, is essential in managing myofascial pain and promoting optimal muscle function.

- A type of secondary trigger point is known as a satellite trigger point. The distinction between satellite and secondary trigger points lies in their location and relationship to the primary trigger point. Satellite trigger points are smaller points that occur near the primary trigger point and are often situated in muscles that work together or are functionally linked to the muscles housing the primary trigger points. They form as a result of the referred pain and dysfunction generated by the primary trigger point, creating a cluster of interconnected trigger points that contribute to the overall discomfort experienced by the individual. In contrast, secondary trigger points typically refer to trigger points that develop in muscles separate and distinct from the muscles containing the primary trigger points. While they remain related to the presence of the primary trigger point, they are not located directly adjacent to it like the satellite trigger points.

ii) Latent trigger Points

- Latent trigger points are specific types (of trigger points) that typically do not cause pain or discomfort in normal circumstances, hence the term latent. Unlike active trigger points, which are responsible for referring pain and other symptoms, latent trigger points remain inactive and do not manifest noticeable sensations until they are activated.[1] As a result, individuals may be unaware of their existence until certain factors or triggers cause them to become active, leading to the onset of pain or discomfort.

- Despite their dormant nature, latent trigger points can play a significant role in developing myofascial pain syndrome and other musculoskeletal conditions. These trigger points may remain latent and undetected until a physical examination or specific triggers, such as stress, injury, or overuse, activate them. Once activated, latent trigger points can transition into active trigger points, contributing to pain, limited range of motion, and related symptoms.

Indications for Treating Trigger Points

- **Localised pain**: Trigger points typically generate pain in a specific area of varying intensity and are often described as aching, throbbing, or sharp. This pain is often deep within the muscle and exacerbated by movement or pressure.

  Myofascial pain syndrome (MPS) is a condition characterized by chronic pain in the musculoskeletal system. MPS is typified by the presence of trigger points in the muscles or fascia, which can lead to persistent pain and discomfort. Myofascial pain is typically described as a deep, aching, or persistent pain that originates from specific points in muscles or the surrounding connective tissue (fascia). This pain is often localized to the area where trigger points are present.

- **Palpable muscle knots**: Trigger points are taut bands or nodules which can be felt within the muscle tissue when trigger points are present. These firm knots or tight bands can be detected through palpation and are typically tender or sensitive to touch.

- **Restricted range of motion**: Trigger points can cause muscle stiffness and limit the ability to move the affected muscle fully.

- **Muscle weakness**: In some conditions, trigger points can induce muscle weakness or a sense of fatigue in the affected area. The associated muscle may also feel weaker than usual, making performing tasks requiring strength or endurance challenging.

- **Referred pain**: Trigger points can cause referred pain, which means pain is experienced in a different body area from where the trigger point is located. For example, a trigger point in the upper back might elicit pain radiating down the arm or into the chest area. These could be secondary trigger points or satellite trigger points.

- **Muscle twitching or spasms**: Trigger points can occasionally provoke involuntary muscle twitches or spasms. These sudden, brief contractions of the muscle fibres may be visible or felt as uncomfortable or painful jerking movements.

- **Sensitivity to applied pressure**: Applying pressure to a trigger point can evoke a localised response, known as a "twitch response." This response is a distinguishing characteristic of trigger points, and pressing on the trigger point may reproduce the associated pain and discomfort.

Explanation of Mechanisms of Trigger Point Therapy

- The Pain Gate Control Theory may explain how trigger point therapy can alleviate pain. According to this theory, pain signals travel through nerve fibres from the body to the brain. The theory suggests that there is a "gate" in the spinal cord that can either allow or block the transmission of these pain signals.[2] Different types of nerve fibres, large-diameter sensory fibres and small-diameter pain fibres regulate this gate. When the large sensory fibres are stimulated, such as through pressure or touch, they have the ability to "close" the gate and prevent the transmission of pain signals from the small pain fibres. When stimulated or pressure is applied to the trigger point, the large sensory fibres may get stimulated, leading to closing the gate and inhibiting pain signal transmission.

By interfering with the transmission of pain signals to the brain, trigger point therapy may relieve pain or reduce pain perception.[3] Activating the large sensory fibres through trigger point therapy essentially overrides the pain signals sent by the small pain fibres, resulting in relief and improved comfort.

Gate Control Theory of Pain

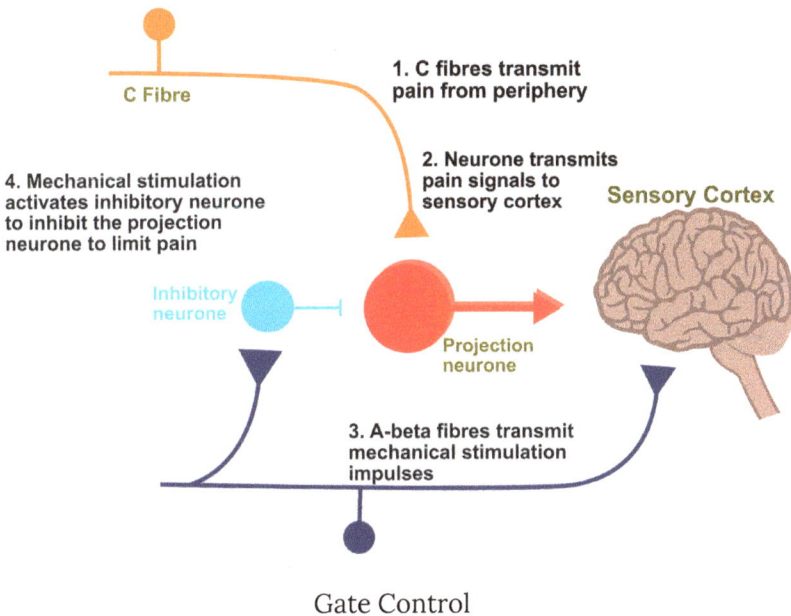

C Fibre

1. C fibres transmit pain from periphery

4. Mechanical stimulation activates inhibitory neurone to inhibit the projection neurone to limit pain

2. Neurone transmits pain signals to sensory cortex

Sensory Cortex

Inhibitory neurone

Projection neurone

3. A-beta fibres transmit mechanical stimulation impulses

Gate Control

- Trigger point therapy may modulate the response of the nervous system to pain. Stimulation of trigger points may initiate a series of neurological responses, including the release of neurotransmitters and neuromodulators. These substances can influence pain receptors, alter the transmission of nerve signals, and impact pain perception, ultimately leading to pain relief.[4]

- Trigger point therapy may enhance blood circulation to the affected area. Improved blood circulation brings oxygen, nutrients, and immune cells to the area, promoting tissue healing and so reducing muscle tension.

- The manipulation of trigger points may stimulate the release of various neurochemicals in the body, such as endorphins, which are natural pain-relieving and mood-enhancing substances. Endorphins bind to opioid receptors in the brain and spinal cord, reducing pain perception and generating a sense of well-being.[5]

- When pressure is applied to trigger points, muscle tension is released, enabling the elongation and relaxation of the muscle fibres. This relaxation helps alleviate muscle spasms, reduce stiffness, and improve overall muscle function.[6]

- Treating trigger points may have structural and mechanical effects on the tissue by breaking up adhesions or knots within muscle fibres, enhancing tissue mobility and restoring proper alignment of muscle fibres, fascia, and other connective tissues.[7]

- Inserting a needle in proximity of motor endplates, the points where nerve signals communicate with muscle fibres, has the potential to induce depolarization of these endplates. This depolarization process triggers the release of acetylcholine, a neurotransmitter crucial for muscle contractions. The consequent relaxation of muscle fibres can effectively relieve tension within the trigger point.[8]

Locating Trigger Points

Trigger points often have characteristic pain patterns associated with them. These pain patterns can involve local pain at the site of the trigger point and referred pain in distant areas.

Various manual palpation techniques can be used to assess the muscles and identify trigger points. These techniques include static compression, rolling or gliding, pinching, or stretching the muscle fibres. The affected muscle is palpated systematically, applying steady pressure and observing the patient's response to identify tender or taut areas that may indicate trigger points. A local muscle twitch or jump response can occur when palpating a trigger point. This involuntary muscle contraction can confirm the presence of an active trigger point.

A step-by-step guide to locating trigger points

Before beginning, it is important to understand the symptoms described by the patient experiencing pain or discomfort. Common indications of trigger points include localised pain, tenderness, and referred pain.

Patient Background

- Start by gathering a comprehensive history from the patient, including details about their pain patterns and activities that affect it. From this information, identify the muscle affected. Observe the patient's posture and movements for signs of muscle imbalances or tension that might point to trigger points.

Manual Palpation Method

- Using fingertips, thumbs, or the tips of hands, feel the muscle groups in the affected area. Gradually increase pressure as you palpate to detect any areas of tightness, tenderness, or resistance. Note any changes in muscle texture. Trigger points can feel like knots or tight bands embedded in the muscle tissue.

Taut Bands

- Search for taut bands or cords within the muscle, which are often present when trigger points exist. Firmly press or compress the suspected trigger point, observing whether it reproduces the patient's usual pain. Ensure the patient's reported pain aligns with common referral patterns associated with the muscle under examination. If pain or tenderness is felt when pressure is applied, you might have located a trigger point. Perform repeated assessment, as trigger points typically yield consistent pain or discomfort upon pressure. Observe any involuntary muscle twitch, as this is a reliable indicator of trigger points.

Referral Pain Pattern

- Ask the patient if they experience discomfort or pain radiating to other areas when you apply pressure to specific points as this may indicate secondary or satellite trigger points.

Muscle Assessment

- Evaluate the condition of the muscle surrounding the trigger point noting any muscle tension, tightness, or changes in muscle texture. Palpate adjacent areas as well to identify any secondary or satellite trigger points that may contribute to the overall pain pattern. *See the section below on Functional Palpitation.*

Trigger Point Referral Charts

- Use trigger point referral charts or maps that illustrate the common referral patterns associated with specific trigger points. These charts can provide valuable guidance in identifying trigger points based on the patient's reported symptoms and location. Although convenient and relatively simple way to identify trigger point, this method should be used as a guide only.

Needle Insertion Technique

Once trigger point/s are identified, insert a fine filament needle (acupuncture needle) into the muscle tissue. The needle is typically inserted to a depth that reaches the trigger point or taut band. The insertion should be quick. A key feature of dry needling is eliciting a local twitch response (LTR). When the needle is inserted into the trigger point, it can cause a characteristic involuntary twitch or contraction of the muscle. The LTR is a reflexive response that occurs due to the stimulation of the muscle spindle fibres within the trigger point. The LTR is believed to help release tension in the muscle, decrease pain, and promote muscle relaxation.

From a practical point of view, when an acupuncture needle is inserted into a muscle, the feel of the needle may change from a smooth glide to a somewhat firmer feel as the needle penetrates the muscle.

Dry needling techniques can vary based on the practitioner's training, approach, and the treated muscle. Some standard techniques include:

- **Pistoning**: This technique moves the needle in and out of the trigger point rhythmically, typically with small up-and-down movements.

- **Twisting**: The needle is gently twisted or rotated while inserted into the muscle to enhance the therapeutic effect. The practitioner should be aware of the "stuck needle" effect, which can arise due to the contraction of the muscle fibre which firmly holds the needle.

- **Periosteal pecking**: Involves using an acupuncture needle to actually peck at the bone in an attempt to help with healing (Dunning et al, 2018). It involves administering a sequence of swift and deliberate taps, to a particular region of a bone, particularly in proximity to the outer layer where the periosteum, envelopes the bone. Through these rapid and controlled taps, the practitioner aims to activate the area and facilitate relaxation, thereby alleviating tension in the connected muscle.

The insertion of the needle depends on the muscle being treated. Sometimes, the needle may be inserted to a deeper level within the muscle tissue to reach deeper trigger points or tight bands. Superficial needling may be used for more superficial muscles or areas where deep needling may not be necessary or appropriate.

Post-Needling Sensation

After treatment, some individuals may experience post-needling sensations. These can include temporary soreness, aching, or a feeling of heaviness or fatigue in the treated area. These sensations typically subside within a short period, but some mild post-treatment soreness may persist for a day or two. To reduce the post-needling effects, patients could be advised to drink more water as the treatment may release toxins which are eliminated.

It is important to note that while trigger point therapy can provide acute pain relief, it may not address the underlying causes of the trigger points or provide long-term resolution.

Functional Palpitation

Functional palpation in trigger point therapy involves an examination of muscles and surrounding tissues while the patient *engages in specific movements*. This method allows the practitioner to assess how trigger points affect actual muscle function, observing movement patterns, feeling for abnormalities, evaluating range of motion, and identifying referral patterns of trigger point pain. By using this approach with other assessment techniques outlined above, the practitioner can gain a comprehensive understanding of how trigger points impact activities and the functioning of the affected muscles.

A step-by-step guide to Functional Palpitation:

- Trigger points within a muscle can cause movement dysfunction or altered movement patterns. For instance, a trigger point in the quadriceps muscle might lead to difficulty in fully extending the knee or performing activities that require strong knee extension, such as jumping or squatting.

- Trigger points can generate pain when the affected muscle is activated or used. For example, a trigger point in the trapezius muscle may cause pain when elevating the shoulders or engaging in shoulder movement activities.

- Trigger points can induce muscle weakness or inhibition. During palpation, the practitioner may observe reduced muscle strength or difficulties contracting the muscle due to the presence of trigger points.

- Trigger points often produce pain in other areas of the body, which can offer clues to their location. For instance, a gluteus minimus muscle trigger point might refer to pain in the hip or the front of the thigh, indicating its presence.

- Trigger points can restrict the range of motion in a muscle or joint. Individuals may experience decreased flexibility or range when attempting to move the muscle associated with the trigger point.

Common Areas of Trigger Points

As trigger points are located around the muscles described below, please refer to the muscles described in earlier chapters (anatomy).

Shoulder Area:

- **Deltoid:** covers the shoulder joint and allows for shoulder abduction, shoulder flexion, shoulder extension, and rotation.

  Trigger Points and Symptoms: Trigger points in the deltoid can cause pain and tenderness around the shoulder and upper arm. Depending on the location of the trigger point, individuals may experience discomfort during arm movements and difficulty with lifting or reaching.

- **Rotator cuff muscles** (Supraspinatus, Infraspinatus, Teres Minor, Subscapularis): A group of four muscles that stabilise the shoulder joint and assist with various movements, including shoulder rotation and elevation.

  Trigger Points and Symptoms: Trigger points in the rotator cuff muscles can lead to pain and tenderness around the shoulder, especially when lifting the arm or performing overhead activities. Individuals may also experience weakness and reduced range of motion in the shoulder.

- **Trapezius:** Large muscle extending from the neck to the upper back and shoulders. It helps control the movement and stability of the shoulder girdle, including shoulder elevation, retraction (pulling the shoulder blades together), and depression (lowering the shoulders).

  Trigger Points and Symptoms: Trigger points in the trapezius can result in pain and discomfort in the upper back, neck, and shoulders. Individuals may experience tension headaches, limited shoulder movement, and aching in the affected areas.

- **Rhomboids:** Two muscles situated between the shoulder blades. They aid in shoulder retraction, helping to bring the shoulder blades together.

Trigger Points and Symptoms: Trigger points in the rhomboids can cause pain and tenderness between the shoulder blades. Individuals may experience discomfort and restricted movement when bringing the shoulder blades together.

- **Latissimus Dorsi**: Large muscle spanning from the lower back to the upper arm. It plays a role in shoulder adduction and extension.

  Trigger Points and Symptoms: Trigger points in the latissimus dorsi can lead to pain and tenderness in the mid-back and shoulder. Individuals may experience discomfort during arm movements, particularly when reaching overhead or across the body.

- **Pectoralis Major:** Large chest muscle that contributes to shoulder flexion and adduction.

  Trigger Points and Symptoms: Trigger points in the pectoralis major can cause pain and tenderness in the chest and front of the shoulder. Individuals may experience discomfort when performing movements involving the shoulder, such as reaching or lifting.

Elbow and Upper Arm:

- **Biceps Brachii:** Commonly known as the biceps, is a two-headed muscle located on the front of the upper arm. Its primary functions include flexing the elbow joint and supinating the forearm (turning the palm upward).

  Trigger Points and Symptoms: Trigger points in the biceps brachii can lead to pain in the front of the shoulder and upper arm. Individuals may experience discomfort when bending the elbow or rotating the forearm, and these trigger points can sometimes contribute to shoulder pain.

- **Triceps Brachii:** A three-headed muscle on the upper arm's back. Its primary role is to extend the elbow joint.

Trigger Points and Symptoms: Trigger points in the triceps brachii can cause pain in the back of the upper arm and shoulder. Individuals may experience discomfort when straightening the elbow or when pressure is applied to the back of the arm.

- **Brachialis:** Located beneath the biceps brachii on the front of the upper arm. It plays a significant role in elbow flexion.

  Trigger Points and Symptoms: Trigger points in the brachialis can cause deep pain in front of the upper arm. Individuals may experience discomfort when bending the elbow, and these trigger points can sometimes be mistaken for biceps tendinitis.

- **Brachioradialis:** Located on the forearm, but it contributes to elbow flexion and forearm pronation (turning the palm downward) when the elbow is flexed.

  Trigger Points and Symptoms: Trigger points in the brachioradialis can cause pain in the forearm near the elbow. Individuals may experience discomfort when flexing or rotating the forearm, these trigger points can sometimes be mistaken for symptoms of lateral epicondylitis.

- **Anconeus:** Small muscle located on the back of the elbow joint. It assists in extending the elbow and stabilising the joint during various movements.

  Trigger Points and Symptoms: Trigger points in the anconeus can cause pain and tenderness on the back of the elbow. Individuals may experience discomfort when straightening the arm; these trigger points can sometimes be mistaken for the symptom of medial epicondylitis.

Wrist and Lower Arm:

- **Flexor Carpi Radialis:** Situated on the palm side of the forearm. It is responsible for wrist flexion (bending the wrist downward) and contributes to wrist abduction (moving the hand away from the body's midline).

Trigger Points and Symptoms: Trigger points in the flexor carpi radialis can cause pain and tenderness on the front of the forearm and near the wrist. Individuals may experience discomfort when bending the wrist or performing gripping activities.

- **Flexor Carpi Ulnaris:** Located on the inner side of the forearm. It plays a role in wrist flexion and adduction (moving the hand toward the body's midline).

  Trigger Points and Symptoms: Trigger points in the flexor carpi ulnaris can lead to pain and tenderness on the inner side of the forearm and near the wrist. Individuals may experience discomfort when bending the wrist or engaging in activities involving ulnar deviation (sideways wrist movement towards the little finger side).

- **Extensor Carpi Radialis Longus and Brevis:** Positioned on the back of the forearm. They are involved in wrist extension (bending the wrist backwards) and contribute to wrist abduction.

  Trigger Points and Symptoms: Trigger points in the extensor carpi radialis muscles can cause pain and tenderness on the back of the forearm and near the wrist. Individuals may experience discomfort when straightening the wrist or performing repetitive gripping activities.

- **Extensor Carpi Ulnaris:** Located on the back of the forearm, opposite the flexor carpi ulnaris. It is responsible for wrist extension and wrist adduction.

  Trigger Points and Symptoms: Trigger points in the extensor carpi ulnaris can lead to pain and tenderness on the back of the forearm and near the wrist. Individuals may experience discomfort when straightening the wrist or performing activities involving radial deviation.

- **Pronator Teres:** Muscle situated on the inner side of the forearm. It is responsible for forearm pronation (turning the palm downward).

  Trigger Points and Symptoms: Trigger points in the pronator teres can cause pain and tenderness on the inner side of the forearm. Individuals may experience discomfort when turning the palm downward or performing repetitive pronation movements.

- **Supinator:** Located on the outer side of the forearm. It is responsible for forearm supination (turning the palm upward).

  Trigger Points and Symptoms: Trigger points in the supinator can lead to pain and tenderness on the outer side of the forearm. Individuals may experience discomfort when turning the palm upward or performing repetitive supination movements.

The Hip Area:

- **Gluteus Maximus:** The most significant muscle in the gluteal group, it extends the hip joint and aids in activities like rising from a seated position, climbing stairs, and running.

  Trigger Points and Symptoms: When trigger points develop in the gluteus maximus, individuals may experience pain and tenderness in the buttocks. The discomfort can also radiate down the back of the thigh and into the lower leg.

- **Gluteus Medius**: Positioned on the lateral side of the hip, the gluteus medius contributes to stabilising the pelvis during walking and other weight-bearing movements. It also assists in hip abduction.

  Trigger Points and Symptoms: Trigger points in the gluteus medius can lead to pain in the hip, buttocks, and the side of the thigh. Additionally, individuals might find it difficult to walk or balance on one leg.

- **Gluteus Minimus:** Situated beneath the gluteus medius, the gluteus minimus aids in hip abduction and internal rotation.

  Trigger Points and Symptoms: Individuals may experience pain in the hip area and the front of the thigh when trigger points develop in the gluteus minimus. Crossing the legs and lying on the affected side might become uncomfortable.

- **Piriformis:** The muscle is deep within the gluteal region and plays a role in external rotation and stabilising the hip joint.

  Trigger Points and Symptoms: Trigger points in the piriformis muscle can lead to piriformis syndrome, wherein the muscle irritate or compress the sciatic nerve. This can result in pain, tingling, or numbness along the back of the leg and possibly extending into the foot.

- **Iliopsoas** (Psoas Major and Iliacus): Formed by the psoas major and iliacus muscles, plays a significant role in hip flexion and is involved in activities like walking, running, and sitting up from a lying position.

  Trigger Points and Symptoms: Trigger points in the iliopsoas muscle can cause deep pain in the front of the hip or groin area. Additionally, individuals may experience lower back discomfort and pain while lifting the knee toward the chest.

- **Tensor Fasciae Latae** (TFL): Assists in hip flexion, abduction, and internal rotation.

  Trigger Points and Symptoms: When trigger points develop in the TFL, individuals may experience pain in the hip and the lateral thigh. They might also feel discomfort while lying on the affected side.

Upper Leg and Knee:

- **Quadriceps** (Quadriceps Femoris): Muscle group consists of four muscles situated on the front of the thigh: Rectus Femoris, Vastus Lateralis, Vastus Medialis, and Vastus Intermedius. They collaborate to extend the knee joint, enabling actions like kicking, walking, and running.

  Trigger Points and Symptoms: When trigger points develop in the quadriceps, individuals may experience pain and tenderness in front of the thigh and around the knee area. Straightening the knee completely might become difficult, and discomfort may arise during activities that engage the quadriceps, such as squatting or climbing stairs.

- **Hamstrings:** Group of three muscles on the back of the thigh: Biceps Femoris, Semitendinosus, and Semimembranosus. They are responsible for knee flexion (bending) and hip extension, aiding in walking, running, and bending over.

  Trigger Points and Symptoms: Trigger points in the hamstrings can cause pain in the back of the thigh and behind the knee. This discomfort may intensify during activities that involve knee flexion, such as prolonged sitting or performing exercises like deadlifts and leg curls.

- **Gastrocnemius** (Calf Muscle): Situated at the back of the lower leg, the gastrocnemius muscle crosses the knee joint and is involved in plantar flexion of the foot. It plays a role in walking and running.

  Trigger Points and Symptoms: Trigger points in the gastrocnemius can lead to calf pain, tightness and potentially contribute to knee pain. Individuals may experience discomfort while walking or standing on tiptoes.

- **Popliteus:** A small muscle located at the back of the knee joint. It assists in unlocking the knee by medially rotating the tibia during the initial phase of knee flexion.

Trigger Points and Symptoms: Trigger points in the popliteus muscle can cause pain and tenderness at the back of the knee. This may result in difficulty with knee flexion or discomfort when squatting or descending stairs.

- **Sartorius:** A long, thin muscle that runs from the front of the hip to the inner side of the knee. It helps in hip flexion, knee flexion, and external rotation of the hip.

  Trigger Points and Symptoms: Trigger points in the sartorius muscle can cause pain and discomfort in the front of the hip, thigh, and knee. Individuals may experience pain when walking, running, or performing hip and knee flexion activities. The pain may also radiate down the inner side of the thigh and can be mistaken for other conditions, such as hip or knee joint issues.

Ankle and Lower Leg Area:

- **Gastrocnemius** (Calf Muscle): Large muscle at the lower leg's back. It is responsible for plantar flexion of the foot, which involves pointing the toes downward. The gastrocnemius actively engages in activities like walking, running, and jumping.

  Trigger Points and Symptoms: Trigger points in the gastrocnemius can result in calf pain, tightness, and restricted ankle movement. These trigger points may cause discomfort while walking or standing on tiptoes.

- **Soleus:** Lies beneath the gastrocnemius and contributes to the foot's plantar flexion. It is particularly active during standing, walking, and running.

  Trigger Points and Symptoms: Trigger points in the soleus can cause deep, aching pain in the calf. People may experience discomfort during activities that engage the soleus, such as prolonged standing or walking.

- **Tibialis Anterior:** Situated on the front of the lower leg and is responsible for dorsiflexion of the foot, which involves lifting the toes upward. It helps control the lowering of the foot during walking and supports the arch of the foot.

  Trigger Points and Symptoms: Trigger points in the tibialis anterior can lead to pain and tenderness in front of the lower leg. These trigger points might cause difficulty in dorsiflexing the foot and discomfort during activities that involve walking or lifting the toes.

- **Peroneus Longus and Peroneus Brevis** (Peroneals): Muscles are located on the outer side of the lower leg and aid in the eversion of the foot, which involves turning the sole outward and stabilising the ankle during walking and running.

  Trigger Points and Symptoms: Trigger points in the Peroneals can cause pain and tenderness on the outer side of the lower leg and around the ankle. These trigger points might lead to difficulties with ankle eversion and discomfort during walking or weight-bearing activities.

- **Tibialis Posterior:** Positioned deep within the calf and plays a crucial role in supporting the foot arch and inverting the foot, that is turning the sole inward.

  Trigger Points and Symptoms: Trigger points in the tibialis posterior can cause pain and tenderness along the inside of the lower leg and ankle. These trigger points might lead to difficulties with foot inversion and discomfort during walking or activities that involve supporting body weight on foot.

Conclusion

Trigger point therapy is a valuable and versatile tool in the treatment of musculoskeletal and sports injuries. Its effectiveness lies in the targeted approach to alleviating pain and dysfunction by addressing specific hyperirritable points within muscle tissue. By releasing tension, improving blood flow, and enhancing muscle function, trigger point therapy can significantly contribute to the rehabilitation and recovery process of the patient whose primary complaint is pain. When used with acupuncture which is used to treat the root cause of the symptoms, the combination of the two therapies provides the TCM practitioner with a very effective therapy to treat sports and musculoskeletal injuries (as long as the practitioner is suitably trained for using trigger point therapy).

References

1. Clinical implication of latent myofascial trigger point; D Celik, EK Mutlu. Current pain and headache reports, 2013.
2. R. Melzack, "Myofascial trigger points: relation to acupuncture and mechanisms of pain," Archives of Physical Medicine and Rehabilitation, vol. 62,1981.
3. García, Carlos M., and María I. M. Fontelles. "Sistemas Cannabinoide Y Opioide En Los Mecanismos Y El Control Del Dolor." Reumatología ClíNica, 2009.
4. J. P. Shah, "Uncovering the biochemical milieu of myofascial trigger points using in vivo microdialysis," Journal of Musculoskeletal Pain, vol. 16, 2008.
5. Research Group of Acupuncture Anesthesia BMC, "Effect of needling positions in acupuncture on pain threshold of human skin," Zhonghua Yi Xue Za Zhi, vol. 3, 1973.
6. B Cagnie, V Dewitte, T Barbe, F Timmermans, N Delrue, M Meeus; Physiologic effects of dry needling. Current pain and headache reports, 2013
7. RD Gerwin, J Dommerholt, JP Shah; An expansion of Simons' integrated hypothesis of trigger point formation. Current pain and headache reports, 2004.
8. Abbaszadeh-Amirdehi ANN, Naghdi S. Nourbakhsh. Neurophysiological and clinical effects of dry needling in patients with upper trapezius myofascial trigger points. MR. J Bodyw Mov Ther. 2017

Chapter 8

Cupping Therapy for Musculoskeletal and Sports Injuries

In recent years, Cupping Therapy has emerged as a popular method for treating musculoskeletal and sports injuries. Cupping's exact origins are not well-documented, but its earliest recorded evidence dates back to ancient Egyptian times, around 1550 BC, in the Ebers Papyrus, one of the oldest medical textbooks in history, which described using cupping therapy for treating various conditions.[1] Cupping therapy also has roots in Traditional Chinese Medicine, which has been practised for thousands of years. The earliest mention of Cupping can be found in the ancient Chinese text called the "Bo Shu" (Book of Mountains and Seas), which dates back to the 4th century BC.

There are two types of cupping therapy, Dry and Hijama or wet cupping.[2] In dry cupping, treatment involves the creation of suction, whereas, with wet cupping, the practitioner carries out controlled medical bleeding and suction. *The text below only refers to Dry Cupping Method.*

Dry Cupping

Dry cupping is a form of therapy that involves creating a vacuum or suction inside a cup, which is then placed on specific areas of the skin. This process is typically achieved using heat or a mechanical pump to remove the air from the cup, creating a vacuum seal. In Traditional Chinese Medicine (TCM), there are two methods of dry cupping; Retaining and Sliding cupping or Myofascial cupping.

Retaining Cup Method

The retaining cup method is a technique of cupping therapy that involves placing cups on specific acupuncture points or other body areas and keeping them in position for a period, typically ranging from a few minutes to up to 20 minutes. The time depending on the condition being treated, body area and the constitution of the patient. The cups used in this method can be made of glass, silicon, or bamboo. The choice of cups may vary depending on the practitioner's preference and the individual's condition.

Based on the individual's unique condition and treatment goals, the practitioner chooses appropriate acupuncture points or specific areas on the body to place the cups, The cup is positioned on the skin's surface, after the air within it is removed to establish a vacuum effect. This suction action causes the skin and the tissues underneath to be gently drawn upwards into the cup, resulting in a raised or lifted appearance of the skin. There are two methods of achieving the vacuum effect;

- Using a mechanical pump in cupping therapy offers a controlled and adjustable method for creating the necessary suction. This helps ensure a safe and effective treatment. The mechanical method is a modern variation of cupping, as traditional methods rely on heat and flame to create the vacuum, as described below.

- Using a flame and cup is a traditional method of cupping therapy that has been practiced for centuries. In this method, a small piece of cotton soaked in medical-grade alcohol is ignited, generating a flame. Once the flame is

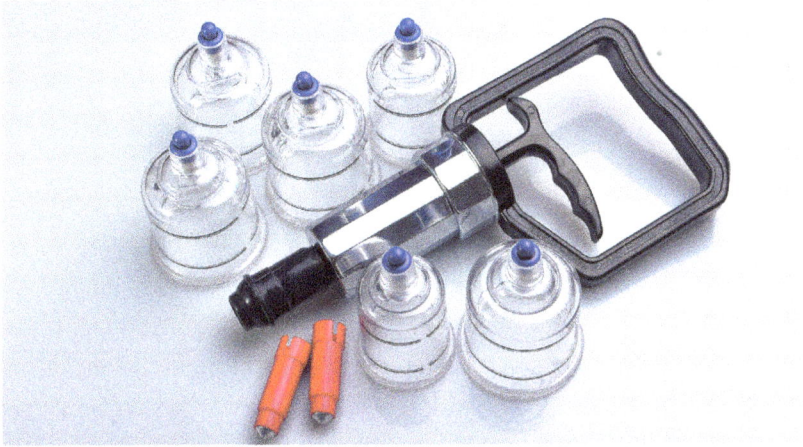

Cupping Pump Set

established, the cotton is placed inside the cup and is swiftly removed. The cup is immediately positioned onto the skin. As the oxygen within the cup is consumed by the flame, a vacuum is formed, leading to the elevation of the

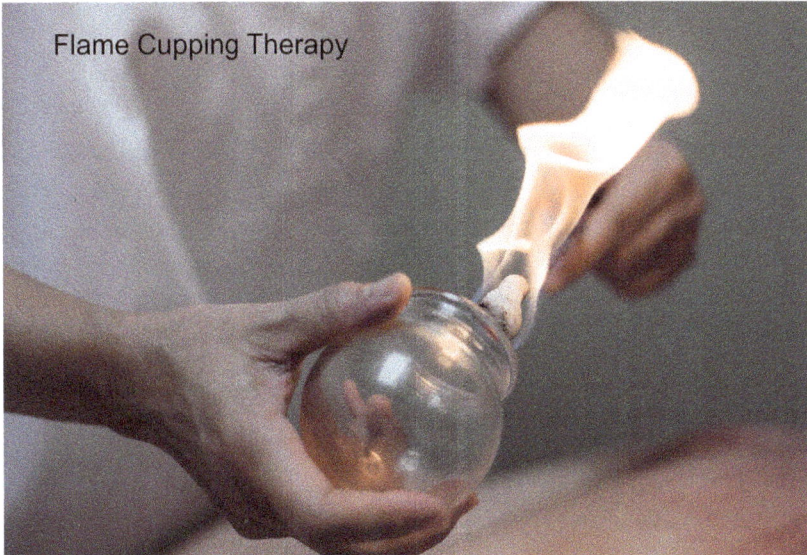

Flame Cupping Therapy

Cupping Flame

skin within the cup. Fire cupping method does carry certain risks, as there is a potential for patients to experience burns. Also, this method lacks precise control over the amount of vacuum generated although with experience this can be overcome.

Therapeutic Benefits of Cupping

The suction produced by the cups has several therapeutic effects. Firstly, it stimulates blood flow to the cupped area. With the enhanced blood flow, facilitates the delivery of nutrients and oxygen, which in turn nurtures tissue repair and rejuvenation, aiding the body's innate healing mechanisms.

- **Qi Activation:** According to TCM principles, the suction of the cups also helps invigorate flow of Qi along the body's meridians. By promoting the smooth movement of Qi, cupping aims to restore balance and harmony within the body, addressing imbalances and blockages that may be contributing to pain or discomfort.

- **Pain Relief:** The retaining cup can relieve pain by releasing muscle tension and reducing spasms in the cupped area. The suction effect helps to stretch and elongate muscle fibres, promoting relaxation and reducing stiffness. As a result, cupping therapy is often used to treat musculoskeletal pain, sports injuries, and other conditions associated with muscle tension.

- **Detoxification:** The application of cups to the skin creates negative pressure, which can draw toxins and metabolic waste products from the underlying tissues towards the surface. This can aid in detoxification and the elimination of waste from the body.

- **Reducing Inflammation:** Cupping therapy is thought to stimulate the release of anti-inflammatory substances, which can help reduce inflammation in the body. This can be particularly beneficial for conditions like arthritis and other inflammatory disorders.

- **Improved Blood Circulation:** The suction created by cupping draws blood to the surface of the skin, which can improve circulation in the treated area. This increased blood flow can enhance the delivery of oxygen and nutrients to tissues, promoting healing.

- **Relaxation and Stress Reduction:** The application of cups on the skin can create a sensation of relaxation and comfort. This physical sensation, combined with the calming environment in which cupping therapy can be performed may help reduce stress levels and promote a sense of well-being.

- **Myofascial Release:** Cupping therapy may help release tension in the fascia, connective tissue that surrounds muscles, nerves, and organs. By applying suction, cupping can stretch and loosen the fascia, potentially improving mobility and reducing pain.

- **Trigger Point Therapy:** Cupping can target specific trigger points, which are tight knots of muscle fibres that can cause referred pain. The suction can help release these trigger points, providing relief from localized pain.

- **Immune System Support:** It is thought that cupping therapy can stimulate the immune system by promoting better circulation and lymphatic drainage. This could potentially enhance the body's ability to fight off infections and illnesses.

- **Scar Tissue Reduction:** Cupping therapy may be used to address scar tissue, as the suction can help break down adhesions and promote the healing process.

- **Respiratory Benefits:** In TCM, cupping is sometimes used to treat respiratory conditions like bronchitis and asthma. It is believed that cupping can help clear phlegm and congestion from the lungs, facilitating easier breathing.

In cupping therapy, the strength of suction can vary, and the practitioner can adjust the intensity based on the patient's condition and treatment goals. Different types of cupping strengths are used to achieve specific therapeutic effects.

- **Light Cupping (Weak)**

  Light cupping involves applying gentle suction to the skin. The cups are placed with minimal pressure, creating a mild pulling sensation on the skin. Light Cupping is used for tonifying Qi and Blood with symptoms of deficiency or stagnation. The effect is removing stagnation and strengthening weak Qi and promoting Blood. Light Cupping can be used when the patient has a chronic Blood or Yin deficiency injury.

  Light cupping is also used for patients who are new to cupping or have a low pain threshold. It can be beneficial for promoting relaxation, improving circulation, and addressing minor muscle tension.

- **Moderate Cupping (Medium)**

  Moderate cupping involves applying a moderate (more than in light cupping) amount of suction. The cups create a pulling sensation on the skin, but the pressure is not overly intense. This strength is commonly used to address muscle tension, improve Blood flow, and promote the flow of Qi within the body. It can also be used for Qi and Blood tonification. It is suitable for treating musculoskeletal conditions with Cold, Damp, and Hot Bi Syndromes.

- **Strong Cupping**

  Strong cupping involves applying strong suction, resulting in a more intense pulling sensation on the skin. This strength is often chosen to address deeper muscle tension, chronic pain, and areas of stagnation or tightness. It can be effective for breaking up adhesions, releasing toxins, and promoting deeper circulation. Strong cupping has more of a draining effect, so it can be comparable to reduction and tonification. It is used for athletes with more vigorous Wei Qi. Strong cupping can be used for conditions such as a frozen shoulder.

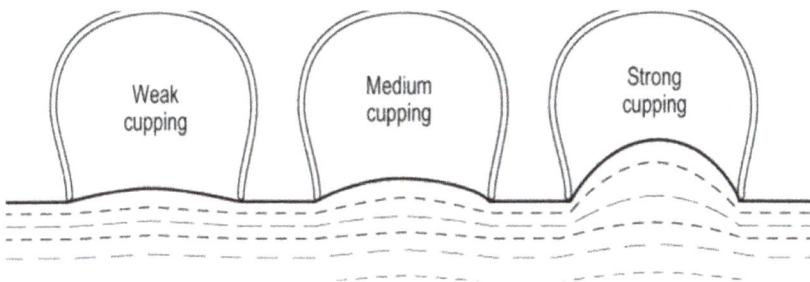

Cupping Strengths

Another version of retaining upping is flash or quick cupping. This method retains cups for a very short period and then removed. This method is useful to tonify and also when there is the presence of pathogenic factors in Bi Syndrome.

Sliding Cup or Myofascial Cupping

With the sliding cup method, as with the retaining cup method, cups made of glass, silicon, or bamboo are placed on the skin. Oil is applied to the skin to facilitate smooth gliding of the cups.

The sliding cup technique involves two primary steps:

- **Cup Placement:** The practitioner selects specific acupuncture points, targeted areas or the meridian affected on the body that requires attention. Once identified, the cups are gently applied to the skin and moved along the meridian or the affected area.

- **Cup Movement:** After securing the cup in place, the practitioner starts moving the cup across the skin's surface. Different techniques, such as linear movements, circular motions, or zigzag patterns, are employed based on the individual's needs and the specific areas being treated.

- As the cups glide over the skin, they create a stretching and pulling effect on the underlying tissues. This action effectively releases adhesions, fascial restrictions, and muscle tightness, resolving myofascial restrictions and promoting increased tissue flexibility. Moreover, the movement of the cups enhances blood circulation and stimulates the lymphatic system, aiding in eliminating metabolic waste and toxins from the tissues.

The sliding cup method is particularly beneficial for addressing issues like muscle pain, stiffness, and localized areas of tension. It is commonly used to alleviate various musculoskeletal conditions, sports injuries, and ailments associated with myofascial pain syndrome.

Post Cupping

The colour changes that appear on the skin after cupping are often considered indicative of the individual's underlying health condition and can help with diagnosis. The specific meanings can vary based on the colour observed. Some common interpretations are:

- Light Red/Pink is indicative of healthy circulation and shows that the treatment has stimulated blood flow in the area and it is considered a positive outcome.

- Bright Red is Qi and or Yin deficiency

- A brownish discoloration indicates older, more chronic issues in the area being treated. It could imply long-standing stagnation or other underlying imbalances.

- A bluish or greenish tinge may indicate the presence of Dampness or Cold in the body. These colours might suggest that the body is working to clear out toxins and address imbalances related to these factors.

- A black or very dark coloration might indicate more severe stagnation, possibly related to very deep-seated issues. It could also suggest an injury or trauma in the area.

Although cupping therapy has been used for centuries in various cultures around the world and has a long history of use, it is important to note that the scientific basis for cupping therapy is still a subject of ongoing research and discussion.

Traditional Chinese Medicine Effects of Cupping Therapy

In Traditional Chinese Medicine, cupping therapy is *thought* to produce the following effects:

- Through the application of suction on the skin, cupping stimulates the flow of Blood and Qi within the meridians, encouraging an improved overall balance and harmony in the body.

- Cupping can be used to eliminate Cold and Damp pathogenic factors, which can cause discomfort or pain by causing stagnation and blockages in the meridians.

- Cupping is frequently used to treat conditions involving Blood Stasis, where blood flow becomes stagnant, potentially resulting in pain, bruising, or swelling. The suction effect of cupping facilitates the dissolution of stagnation, thus supporting better circulation.

- Applying cups to the skin creates negative pressure, drawing toxins and waste products from the underlying tissues towards the surface, where they can be expelled through the skin.

- Cupping can tonify or strengthen Qi and Blood depending on the technique employed. For example, static cupping is associated with tonification, while sliding Cupping may invigorate the flow of Qi and Blood.

- When cupping along meridian lines, the effect will be to "align and relax Qi" in the sliding method. As blockages are cleared, body toxins and pathogenic factors are eliminated, improving tissue healing.

Western Medicine Effects of Cupping

In Western Medicine, cupping therapy is *thought* to produce the following effects:

- The creation of suction by the cups promotes vasodilation, resulting in increased blood flow to the cupped area. This increased blood supply delivers additional oxygen and nutrients to the tissues, aiding healing.

- The increased blood flow and oxygen supply, created by cupping, accelerates tissue repair and regeneration, facilitating the recovery of injured or damaged tissues.

- Cupping therapy can aid in the fragmentation of adhesions and scar tissue that may form post-injury. This enhances tissue flexibility and mobility, so reducing pain and ameliorating the range of motion.

- The suction and stimulation from cupping can activate the immune system, boosting the body's natural defence mechanisms and fostering healing.

- Cupping therapy induces a muscle-relaxing effect, helping to alleviate muscle tension and spasms. This can be particularly beneficial for individuals experiencing muscle-related discomfort, such as those with muscle strains or overuse injuries.

- Neovascularization, also known as angiogenesis, is a biological process in which new blood vessels are formed from existing ones. The process of neovascularization involves specific growth factors and signalling pathways that activate endothelial cells, the building blocks of blood vessels. These endothelial cells then form new capillaries, extending and growing into surrounding tissues, creating a network of blood vessels to supply the newly formed tissue. Neovascularisation occurs in response to blood being drawn in the subdermal area due to the effects of negative pressure caused by cupping, causing microtrauma and separation. The body responds by stimulating an inflammatory response, a natural healing process.

Use of Cupping in Pre and Post Sports Activities

The negative pressure during Cupping creates a "stretch" in the soft tissue and fascia, having the effect of relaxing the muscles. The muscles increase their range of motion and performance in a relaxed state. Due to this effect, cupping can be used as part of the warm-up regime before undertaking physical exercise or participating in a sports activity. The cupping method used is sliding, applied lightly over lower limbs, shoulder area, and lower back. The effect of cupping before an event is to encourage blood and lymph to flow gently (similar to a warm-up exercise). Cupping can also be used after an event. This encourages blood flow so that toxins and waste metabolites from the area are removed, preventing muscle fatigue. However, cupping should not be undertaken if the athlete is suffering from muscle fatigue or an injury.

Contraindications for Cupping

- Injuries in the acute and early subacute phases.
- Skin must be intact, not broken.

- Skin irritation, eczema, psoriasis and moles.
- When skin bruises easily.
- Pregnancy.
- Unhealed fracture.
- Poor circulation.
- Anticoagulants.
- Large superficial blood vessels and varicose veins.
- Post-surgical scars.

Useful areas of Cupping

Both retaining cup or sliding cup method can be used, depending on the presenting symptoms and the muscles affected.

- **Rotator Cuff and Shoulder Injuries** (medium Cupping for 10 minutes)

  Points: LU2, SP20, SI9, SI10, SI11, LI16 and SJ14.

  If the pain radiates to the arm, add LI15, LI14 and SJ13. If the pain radiates to the neck, add SI12

- **Elbow and Wrist** (Light to Medium 10 – 15 minutes)

  No specific point, so use Ah Shi points but with light to medium pressure.

- **Lower Back** (Medium 10 – 15 minutes)

  Points: DU3, BL26 and BL28. If the pain radiates towards the hip area, use DU3, BL53, and BL54.

- **Hip** (Medium 10 – 15 minutes)

  Points: BL28, BL53, GB30 and extra point Guihai

- **Hamstring Injuries** (Medium to Strong)

For hamstring injuries, use sliding techniques: for lateral muscles, the cupping application starts from GB30, moving towards GB32. For medial muscles, the cupping application starts from BL36, moving towards BL40.

- **Quadriceps Injuries** (Light to Medium).

Note: Vastus Medialis is a very sensitive muscle for cupping so warn patient before carrying out cupping.

For quadriceps injuries, use sliding techniques starting from just below ST31 and moving towards ST33. For the medial aspect, start cupping application LIV10 towards LIV9.

- **Knee Injuries** (Light to Medium)

Points:ST35, ST34, GB34 and LIV8

- **Medial Tibial Stress Syndrome** (Medium)

Use sliding cupping to the outer aspect of the tibia, following the line ST36 to just below ST39

- **Gastrocnemius Muscle** (Medium)

Use sliding cupping from;

BL40 moving towards the heel alongside the Tendocalcaneo

GB34 moving along the Gall Bladder channel terminating GB37

SP9 moving towards and ending at SP6

- **Ankle Injuries**

Points: SP5, ST41, BL62, BL60, KID3 and KID8

Conclusion

When used correctly, cupping therapy is safe with many advantages for treating adhesions, fascial tightness and muscle tightness to resolve myofascial restrictions and promote tissue release. When cupping is carried out over meridian pathways, this opens, drains, and clears the meridian so toxins and blockages are cleared. The key to successful treatment is knowing which type of cupping to use, where to use cupping and when to use cupping.

References

1. www.researchgate.net/publication/Cupping Therapy An Alternative Method of Treating Pain.
2. A.M. Al-Bedah, et al. Classification of cupping therapy: a tool for modernization and standardization. J. Compl. Alternative Med.Res, 1 (2016).

Chapter 9

MOXA

Moxibustion, also known commonly as moxa, is a traditional therapy in Chinese Medicine that involves burning dried mugwort (Artemisia vulgaris) on or near specific acupuncture points or body areas. Commonly called moxa, it is derived from the Japanese word "mogusa" or "mokusa," which translates to "burning herb. Moxibustion has a rich and ancient history that dates back thousands of years, forming an essential part of Traditional Chinese Medicine. Its origins can be traced to ancient China and have since spread to other East Asian nations, including Japan, Korea, and Vietnam. The first recorded use of moxa can be found in the ancient Chinese medical text attributed to the legendary Yellow Emperor, Huangdi, around 2600-2000 BCE.[1]

Mugwort is processed into a soft, wool-like substance called moxa, which can take the form of cones and sticks or be placed on an acupuncture needle in a technique called needle moxibustion. This method places the moxa on an acupuncture needle to create a focused and potent therapeutic approach. In this technique, a small cone or moxa ball is affixed to an acupuncture needle's handle. The moxa is ignited, allowing it to burn slowly and produce heat. As the moxa burns, the heat travels down the needle and reaches the acupuncture point, resulting in a localized warming effect. The combination of acupuncture and moxibustion in needle moxibustion enhances the therapeutic benefits. The heat generated by the burning moxa stimulates the acupuncture point, encouraging the flow of Qi and Blood to the targeted area. This targeted approach can be particularly advantageous for conditions requiring more intensive and direct treatment, such as chronic pain or specific musculoskeletal problems.

While moxibustion is a fundamental component of Traditional Chinese Medicine, its effectiveness for addressing various health conditions mentioned above still requires significant scientific evidence.

Use of Moxa for Musculoskeletal and Sports Injuries

Moxibustion can be a valuable therapy for treating musculoskeletal and sports injuries. Its warming properties and ability to improve Qi and Blood circulation make it well-suited for addressing musculoskeletal issues and aiding recovery from sports-related injuries. Moxibustion can relieve pain, reduce inflammation, relax muscles, promote faster healing, and enhance joint mobility. Moxa can be used as part of a comprehensive approach to managing sports injuries when used with other treatments like acupuncture or herbal medicine. Athletes may also use moxibustion before events to warm up muscles and enhance performance, while the post-event application can aid recovery and reduce muscle soreness.

Moxibustion can be beneficial for various musculoskeletal and sports injuries, including:

- Muscle Strains and Sprains: Moxibustion can help to relax and warm the affected muscles, promoting blood circulation and aiding in the healing process.

- Tendonitis and Tendon Injuries: Moxa can be used to stimulate Blood flow and Qi to the affected tendons, potentially assisting in the recovery process.

- Arthritis and Joint Pain: Moxibustion can be applied to points near arthritic joints to help alleviate pain and improve mobility.

- Bruises and Contusions: The warming effect of moxa helps to disperse stagnant Blood and promote quicker healing of bruises and contusions.

- Repetitive Stress Injuries: Moxibustion may be used to address injuries caused by repetitive motions, such as carpal tunnel syndrome or tennis elbow.

- Low Back Pain: Moxa when applied to specific points on the lower back can help to alleviate tension and pain associated with musculoskeletal issues in this area.

Mechanisms of Moxa

- Moxibustion targets acupuncture points, where Qi is believed to accumulate. By applying heat to these points, moxibustion stimulates and regulates flow of Qi.

- Moxibustion generates localized warmth, causing local Blood vessels to expand, thus enhancing Blood circulation. Improved circulation brings nutrients, oxygen, and immune cells, which support tissue repair and diminish inflammation.

- Traditional Chinese Medicine proposes that moxibustion balances Qi by eliminating stagnation and so enhancing flow of Qi and Blood.

- Moxibustion strengthens Yang energy. By enhancing Yang, moxibustion can counteract conditions linked to Cold and Stagnation.

- The warmth created by moxibustion also disperses Cold and Dampness, which cause pain and discomfort.

Moxibustion is applied by two main methods

- **Direct Moxa**

  In this method, traditionally, a lit moxa cone was placed directly on the skin. However, using this method there is a risk of burning the skin. To avoid this, the practitioner is advised to use "stick on" moxa, as this avoids direct skin contact yet provides all the benefit of moxa. Once the patient starts to feel the warmth, the practitioner takes off the cone. An alternative method uses a protective layer, like salt or garlic, positioned between the moxa cone and the skin. A moxa box can also be used. The box contains ignited moxa which is placed on the area to provide heat therapy.

Another approach involves putting the moxa cone onto an acupuncture needle and lighting it. The moxa burns along the length of the needle until it is completely burnt out. The generated heat travels through the needle, conveying warmth to the acupuncture point.

As the direct method may potentially cause scarring or blistering of the skin, the use of moxa should not be used on the following areas of the body:[2]

- Face.

- Breasts.

- Genitals.

- Major tendons.

- Major creases in the skin.

- Areas close to large blood vessels

Direct moxibustion is less commonly used than indirect moxibustion due to the increased risk of burns and discomfort associated with direct contact between moxa and the skin. However, if used safely and correctly applied, it is beneficial for localized pain relief, such as joint pain, muscle pain, and injuries, as well as chronic and persistent conditions requiring more robust and more direct stimulation.

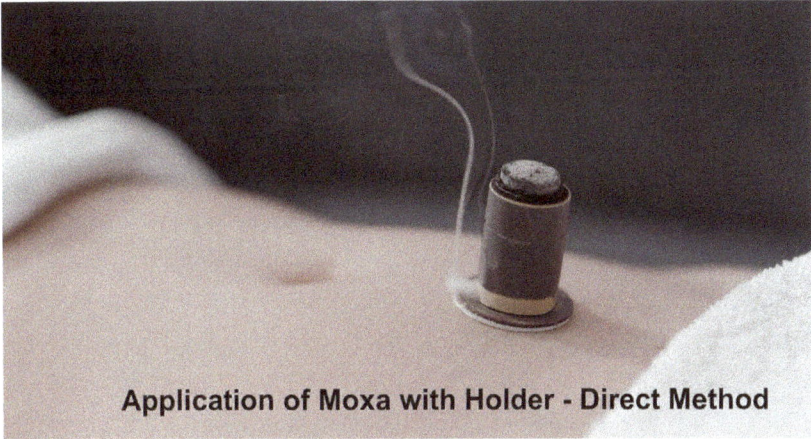

Application of Moxa with Holder - Direct Method

Moxa Direct

- **Indirect Moxa**

  In situations where a moxa cone cannot be used, a moxa stick can be a suitable alternative. The moxa stick is particularly useful for areas where moxa cones may be in a

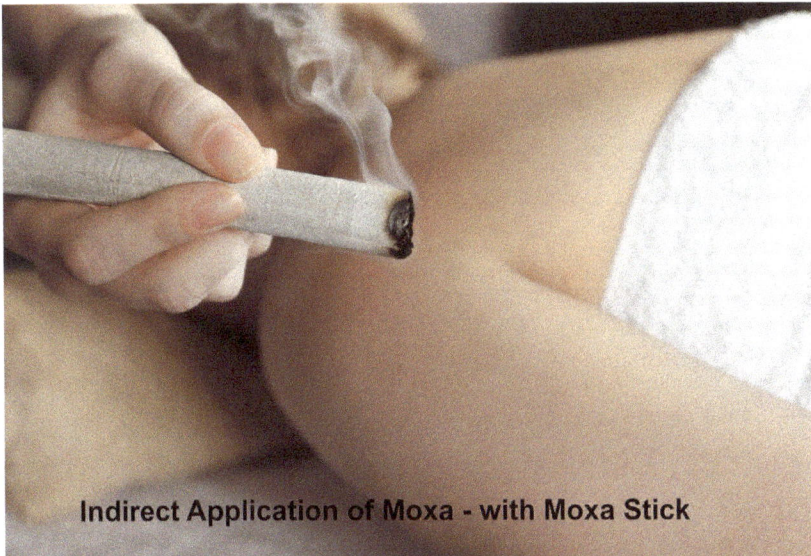

Indirect Application of Moxa - with Moxa Stick

Moxa Stick

challenging position, such as curved surfaces or places that are difficult to access. Unlike moxa cones, moxa sticks can be positioned at varying distances from the skin's surface, allowing for greater control over the heat intensity.

The moxa stick is moved in small circular motions or gentle strokes around the acupuncture point or the area of the body which is being treated. The moxa stick is kept in motion to avoid concentrated heat in one spot.

Common Acupuncture Points used with Moxa

The Shoulder

- **GB21:** Primary point for addressing shoulder pain, tension, and discomfort.

- **LI14:** Alleviates pain and promote circulation in the upper arm.

- **LI15:** Shoulder pain, stiffness, and upper arm issues.

- **SI11:** Shoulder and upper arm pain, particularly related to the rotator cuff muscles.

- **PC6:** Alleviate pain and tension in the upper arm and shoulder by promoting circulation.

- **SI13:** Pain and stiffness in the upper arm and shoulder.

The Elbow

- **LI11:** Primary point for addressing elbow pain, inflammation, and discomfort.

- **TB5:** Alleviate pain and tension in the lower arm and wrist.

- **LI5:** Pain and discomfort in the lower arm and wrist area.

- **PC3:** Promote circulation and alleviate pain in the elbow and lower arm.

- **PC6:** Alleviate pain and tension in the lower arm and wrist by promoting circulation.
- **LI4:** Pain and discomfort in the lower arm and wrist.
- **PC4:** Promote circulation and alleviate pain in the lower arm.

The Wrist

- **LI5:** wrist pain, inflammation, and discomfort.
- **TB5:** Alleviate pain and tension in the wrist.
- **LI6:** Promote circulation and alleviate wrist pain.
- **PC7:** Pain and discomfort in the wrist area.
- **PC6:** Promote circulation and alleviate pain in the wrist.
- **SI3:** Wrist pain and discomfort.
- **GB34:** Promote circulation and alleviate pain in various areas of the body, including the wrist.

The Hip Area

- **GB30** - General hip pain, sciatica, and muscle tension in the hip area.
- **BL57** - Hip and lower back pain, as well as issues related to the gluteal muscles.
- **BL40** - Hip pain, especially if the pain radiates down the leg.
- **BL60** - Pain in the hip, lower back, and leg.
- **GB34** - Hip pain, as well as knee pain and musculoskeletal issues in the leg.
- **LIV8** - Pain and "tension" in the upper leg and thigh area.
- **GB21** - Pain and "tension" in the upper back and upper arm area, which might contribute to upper leg discomfort.

Knee Points

- **ST35**: Knee pain, swelling, and stiffness.
- **EX-LE5** is positioned on the knee joint line, directly on the lateral side of the knee and is used for knee pain and general discomfort, especially on the outer part of the knee.
- **ST34**: Knee pain, inflammation, and other issues related to the quadriceps muscles.
- **GB34**: Knee, as well as hip and leg pain.
- **SP10**: Promote circulation, reduce swelling, and address knee pain.
- **SP9**: Knee pain, swelling, and issues related to the inner thigh muscles.
- **ST36**: Supports overall circulation, beneficial for knee injuries as well as improving circulation and flow of Qi in the entire leg.

Ankle Joint

- **BL60**: Ankle pain, Achilles tendon issues, and foot discomfort.
- **KID3**: Nourishes and tonifies the kidneys, which can be beneficial for lower leg and foot health.
- **ST36**: has been already discussed.
- **GB34**: has been already discussed.
- **SP6**: Promote circulation, relieve pain, and support the overall function of the lower leg and foot.

Benefits of Moxibustion

- Moxibustion's warming sensation can alleviate pain and discomfort associated with musculoskeletal injuries like sprains, strains, and overuse injuries.

- The heat generated by moxibustion can enhance Blood circulation and lymphatic flow in the affected areas, facilitating the delivery of essential nutrients and oxygen, thereby promoting healing.

- Using moxa relaxes muscles and reduces muscle tension and spasms, commonly experienced in sports injuries.

- Moxa can contribute to faster recovery from musculoskeletal injuries by stimulating a more efficient healing response.

- Compared to acupuncture, moxibustion is non-invasive and generally safe when administered correctly.

- Moxibustion can also serve as a preventive measure by strengthening and maintaining the musculoskeletal system, thereby reducing the risk of future sports-related injuries.

Disadvantages of Moxibustion:

- The burning of moxa on or near the skin can pose a risk of burns or skin irritation, if not performed cautiously.

- The burning moxa emits smoke and a distinct odour, which some individuals may find unpleasant.

- Moxibustion may not be suitable for certain health conditions such as skin disorders, and its effectiveness can vary depending on individual cases.

- Some individuals may have sensitivities or allergies to mugwort or other components of moxa, leading to adverse reactions.

Conclusion

Moxibustion's main function is its ability to address pain, inflammation, and resolve circulatory issues, all elements which are useful in the recovery process of musculoskeletal and sports injuries. By applying localized heat to enhance blood circulation to the affected areas, this encourages the delivery of oxygen and essential nutrients necessary for tissue repair and rejuvenation. Furthermore, the relaxing and soothing effects of moxibustion can help alleviate muscle tension, supporting a more comprehensive approach to healing.

References

1. Moxibustion in Early Chinese Medicine and Its Relation to the Origin of Meridians: A Study on the Unearthed Literatures. Published online 2017 Feb 19
2. Moxibustion: Uses, safety, and how to perform.www:medical newstoday.com/articles/what-is-moxibustion

Chapter 10

Traditional Chinese Medicine Medical History Taking and Physical Examination

A patient's detailed medical history is essential to providing safe, effective, and patient-centred care. By discovering a patient's past medical history, current symptoms, and lifestyle factors, the practitioner can gain insights into the individual's health. This information can also assist in the early detection of potential risks, identifying underlying conditions, and establishing accurate diagnoses. Furthermore, understanding a patient's medical history facilitates the implementation of personalized treatment plans tailored to address specific needs and preferences. Beyond its diagnostic use, the history-taking process also promotes a strong patient-practitioner rapport, enhancing communication and trust.

Information Gathered When Taking a Medical History

- **Personal Details:** This should include name, date of birth, address, telephone number and email. Doctor's name and address and next of kin details. Consent for treatment, including permission to contact the patient's doctor.

- **Presenting Complaint:** The presenting complaint is the primary reason a patient seeks treatment. Patients may present with multiple symptoms, but the presenting complaint helps the practitioner prioritize the symptoms causing the most significant discomfort or distress. This allows for a more targeted approach to treatment, addressing the most pressing issues first.

- **Medical History:** Details about the patient's past illnesses, surgeries, injuries, and any chronic or long-standing health conditions they have experienced. This should also include any medications the patient is taking, both oral and topical, as this may have a bearing on the TCM treatment. For example, if a patient is on warfarin, this could cause excessive bleeding when using acupuncture needle, especially if a blood vessel is accidentally punctured.

- **Family History:** Information about the health conditions of the patient's family members, particularly those with hereditary or genetic relevance.

- **Lifestyle and Habits:** Questions about the patient's daily routine, exercise habits, diet, sleep patterns, work environment, and other lifestyle factors that could impact their health. In TCM, lifestyle choices and daily routines in diagnosis and treatment are of immense significance. This impacts the flow of Qi and Blood within the body, thereby directly influencing equilibrium and potential imbalances, dictating whether imbalances manifest as excess, deficiency, stagnation, or patterns of disharmony. The principle of attaining harmony between Yin and Yang is intrinsically linked to lifestyle elements like sleep, exercise routines, and dietary preferences.

- **Emotional Health:** With TCM diagnosis, emotions are crucial to overall health. Enquire about the patient's emotional state, stress levels, and any emotional imbalances they may face. Various emotions are connected to distinct organs and meridians within the context of Traditional Chinese Medicine. For instance, the Liver is associated with anger, the Lungs with sadness, the Spleen with worry, the Kidneys with fear, and the Heart with joy.

Disruptions in emotions can interfere with the smooth circulation of Qi and Blood, which might result in physical manifestations. The evaluation of emotions assists in recognizing the meridians and organs that these disturbances may influence.

- **Digestive Health:** Information about the patient's digestion, bowel movements, appetite, and related symptoms are essential in TCM diagnosis. Digestion is a process that converts food into Qi and Blood, which is crucial for nourishment. The effectiveness of digestion impacts the body's ability to create and distribute these essential energies. Disruptions in digestion can lead to imbalances in the distribution of Qi and Blood, thus affecting various bodily functions. Central to this diagnostic consideration is the Spleen and Stomach, The Spleen facilitates the transformation of nourishment into nutrients, while the Stomach processes and allocates these nutrients. Diagnosing a patient's digestive habits provides valuable insights into the equilibrium or disharmony within these organs, informing the diagnostic process. Furthermore, issues arising from compromised digestion, such as the accumulation of dampness and phlegm, disrupt the smooth flow of Qi, potentially causing a range of health concerns.

- **Menstrual and Reproductive Health:** For female patients, information about menstrual cycles, any gynaecological issues, and reproductive history can be indicative of an underlying disorder, as below;

    - The colour of the menstrual blood is indicative of a number conditions; Bright red signifies excess Yang or Heat, whereas darker hues suggest Blood Stagnation or Cold. Pale or thin blood might point to deficiencies.

    - The presence of clots reflects potential Blood Stasis or compromised circulation.

- Thin, watery blood could indicate Blood Deficiency, while thicker textures may be indicative of Dampness or Phlegm.

- Light or minimal flow may be connected to Blood Deficiency or Cold conditions.

- An abundance of menstrual flow could be associated with excess Yang, Heat, or Blood Stagnation.

- Pain during menstruation relates to Qi Stagnation, Blood Stagnation, or Cold imbalances.

- Emotional fluctuations like mood swings, irritability, or sadness are reflective of Liver energy imbalances which can affect Qi and Blood flow.

• **Urinary and Excretory Function:** Inquiring about urine and bowel habits can provide insights into the body's internal balance. As proper urinary and bowel functions are essential for eliminating waste products, toxins, and excess substances from the body, irregularities in these functions might indicate stagnation or deficiency of Qi and Blood, contributing to various health issues. Abnormal functioning may also indicate imbalances in organ function. For example, changes in bowel habits, such as diarrhoea or constipation, may indicate an imbalance of the Spleen and Stomach organs, as these organs are responsible for proper digestion and absorption of nutrients. Similarly, urinary habits are closely related to Kidney health, and changes in urination patterns can indicate imbalances in Kidney Qi and Yin-Yang, as Kidneys are a vital organ responsible for storing Jing and governing water metabolism.

• **Sleep Patterns:** Specific night-time hours, in a concept called "Organ Clock" or Meridian Clock" correspond to distinct organ systems, aiding in identifying potential imbalances or areas of stress. Accordingly, each organ has two hours of maximum activity and influence during a 24-hour day. These hours correspond to the times when the organ's energy is at its peak and when imbalances or symptoms related to that organ might manifest more prominently. For example, the Liver is believed to be most active from 1 a.m. to 3 a.m. Disruptions during this time might indicate issues related to the Liver's functions, including detoxification, blood regulation, and emotional balance.

- **Observation:** The practitioner should observe the injured area to note any visible signs of injury, such as swelling, bruising, redness, or deformities—observing the surrounding muscles and joints for any changes in shape or alignment. The patient's posture, gait, and movements are assessed to identify compensatory patterns or abnormal biomechanics that might contribute to the injury.

TCM Physical Examination

- **Pulse Diagnosis:** Pulse-taking is a fundamental part of TCM diagnosis. The practitioner assesses both wrists' pulse quality, rate, and rhythm. Pulse diagnosis has a central role in TCM by indicating an understanding of the internal well-being of a patient as the pulse reflects the balance between Yin and Yang and the flow of Qi and Blood. Imbalances in these "energies" can lead to various health issues. Pulse diagnosis helps TCM practitioner to identify these imbalances. Through its analysis, Pulse diagnosis deciphers these imbalances, creating a pathway for targeted interventions to reinstate equilibrium. As healing progresses, pulse diagnosis monitors the change and adapts treatment approaches. Additionally, pulse diagnosis can function for early detection of shifts prior to symptom onset. When integrated with other diagnostic methods, such as tongue, pulse diagnosis constructs a holistic portrait of patients.

Pulse Pattern	Interpretations
Floating Pulse	Exterior condition, Wind or Cold invasion, early stages of illness.
Sinking Pulse	Interior condition, deficiency or excess of Yin, Cold or chronic conditions.
Slippery Pulse	Excess condition, presence of phlegm, dampness, or food stagnation.
Choppy/Wiry Pulse	Stagnation of Qi and Blood, emotional stress or Liver Imbalance.
Thin Pulse	Deficiency condition, Qi or Blood deficiency, Yin deficiency.
Full/Wide Pulse	Excess condition, excess Heat or excess Yang, fevers or acute inflammation.
Empty Pulse	Deficiency condition, Qi, Blood, or Yin deficiency, overall weakness,
Weak Pulse	Deficiency condition, Qi, Blood or Yang deficiency, lack of Qi.
Rapid Pulse	Heat or Excess Yang, fevers, acute inflammation.
Slow Pulse	Cold or Yang deficiency, chronic conditions, weak metabolism.
Hasty/Surging Pulse	Excess condition, emotional imbalance, Liver Qi stagnation, emotional stress.
Knotted/ intermittent Pulse	Blood stagnation, irregular circulation, pain, blockages

Table to Show Pulses and their Indications

Tongue Characteristic	TCM Interpretation
Pale Tongue	Deficiency of Qi or Blood, Cold Syndrome
Red Tongue	Heat, Excess Yang
Purple Tongue	Blood Stagnation
Swollen Tongue	Dampness or Phlegm
Thin Coating	Deficiency or Yin Deficiency
Thick Coating	Excess or Dampness
Yellow Coating	Heat or Infection
White Coating	Cold or Dampness
Cracked Tongue	Yin Deficiency, Heat
Scalloped Edges	Spleen Qi Deficiency, Dampness
Toothmarks on Tongue	Spleen Qi Deficiency
Red Tip of Tongue	Heat in the Heart or Stomach
Pale Swollen Tongue	Spleen or Yang Deficiency
Deep Midline Crack	Stomach Yin Deficiency
Deviated Tongue	Wind Stroke
Pale Purple Tongue	Blood Stagnation with Deficiency
Thin White Coating	Deficiency with Cold
Thick Yellow Coating	Heat with Dampness

Table to Show Tongue Patterns.

- **Tongue Examination**: The tongue also plays a fundamental role in TCM as a diagnostic tool offering insights into an individual's internal health. The tongue's significance in TCM diagnosis is important as the tongue is a visual reflection of the body's internal state. This is indicated by colour, shape, coating, and other features that show imbalances and disharmonies within the body. The tongue's role also extends to early detection, monitoring progress over time, tailoring treatments, revealing constitutional aspects when integrating with other diagnostic methods.

Palpation: Palpation is a crucial part of the examination. The practitioner should use hands to palpate the affected area, assess the condition of the muscles, tendons, ligaments, and bones, checking for tenderness, tension, warmth, or coolness in the injured region. This provides information about the nature and severity of the injury.

Muscle Strength Testing: Examine the strength of the muscles around the injured area. Weakness or imbalances in muscle strength can indicate underlying issues contributing to the injury, such as muscle strains or imbalances in the surrounding structures.

Assessment of Acupuncture Channels and Meridians: As Qi flows through channels or meridians, by palpating along meridians, areas of Qi blockages or imbalances that could be affecting the injured area's healing process can be identified. The assessment of pain along the meridian is also indicative of the meridian/s affected.

Acupuncture Points: Certain acupuncture points act as diagnostic markers, reflecting imbalances in corresponding organs. These points, known as "diagnostic points," exhibit heightened sensitivity or responsiveness in the presence of disruptions along specific meridians. By observing reactions at these points, insights into the state of the meridians and their associated organs can be obtained. Some commonly used diagnostic points are:

- **LU9:** This point on the Lung meridian is often sensitive to Lung-related imbalances, such as respiratory issues, coughing, and skin conditions. It can also indicate imbalances in the Large Intestine meridian.

- **HT3:** Found on the Heart meridian, this point can offer insights into Heart-related imbalances, including palpitations, anxiety, and sleep disturbances.

- **ST36:** Located on the Stomach meridian, ST36 is sensitive to digestive disorders, fatigue, and issues related to the Spleen and Stomach.

- **SP3:** On the Spleen meridian, this point can reflect imbalances in the Spleen, such as digestive problems, weak immunity, and fluid retention.

- **LI4:** This point on the Large Intestine meridian is known for its general sensitivity. It can indicate imbalances related to the Large Intestine and systemic issues like headaches and pain.

- **GB34:** Situated on the Gallbladder meridian, GB34 can offer insights into imbalances affecting the Gallbladder and conditions like joint pain and emotional disturbances.

- **LIV3:** Found on the Liver meridian, LIV3 is sensitive to Liver-related imbalances, including stress, mood swings, and menstrual issues.

- **KID3:** Located on the Kidney meridian, KID3 can reflect imbalances in the Kidneys, as well as issues related to energy levels, reproductive health, and bone health.

- **UB66:** On the Urinary Bladder meridian, this point can indicate imbalances in the Urinary Bladder and issues related to the back and lower body.

- **CV12:** Situated on the Conception Vessel meridian, CV12 is often sensitive to digestive issues and imbalances affecting the Stomach and Spleen.

The Significance of Measuring the Range of Motion

Measuring the range of motion (ROM) is essential for diagnosing musculoskeletal and sports injuries from both Traditional Chinese Medicine and Western Medicine perspectives. The range of motion refers to the degree of movement a joint can achieve in various directions. It is a vital aspect of the physical examination for these injuries.

TCM Perspective

In Traditional Chinese Medicine, the body is perceived as a network of interconnected channels or meridians, facilitating the flow of Qi and Blood. Maintaining a harmonious Qi and Blood flow is crucial for overall health, and disruptions or stagnations within these pathways can result in pain and illness. In cases of injury or imbalance, such stagnation can manifest as pain, swelling, and reduced range of motion.

By assessing the range of motion, TCM practitioners can gauge the Qi and Blood flow within the affected joint, body area or the meridian affected. A limited range of motion may indicate energy blockages or imbalances that require attention. For instance, a joint with decreased flexibility and painful movement could signify Qi and Blood Stagnation along the associated meridian. Recognizing these stagnation patterns enables TCM practitioners to devise treatment strategies, such as acupuncture, cupping, or herbal medicine, to restore the proper flow of Qi and Blood, facilitate healing, and alleviate pain.

Western Medicine Perspective

In Western medicine, evaluating the range of motion is a fundamental aspect of the physical examination for musculoskeletal and sports injuries. This process aids in diagnosing the extent and severity of the injury while identifying the specific structures involved. The range of motion is assessed by examining the joint's movement in various directions and comparing it to its expected normal range. Thus, a limited range of motion in a joint may suggest joint inflammation, ligament injury, muscle strain, or joint capsule contracture. Conversely, an increased range of motion beyond the normal limits might indicate joint instability, dislocation, or ligament laxity. By assessing the range of motion, healthcare professionals can narrow potential diagnoses and guide further diagnostic tests, such as X-rays, MRI, or ultrasound, to confirm the specific injury.

Range of Motion Measurement

A goniometer is a handy tool to measure and assess the range of motion of various body parts. It is a simple device, similar to a protector, which provides precise and objective measurements, allowing the practitioner to quantify the degrees of joint movement in various directions. The device follows standardized protocols, ensuring assessment consistency and enabling better comparison of measurements over time. By identifying limitations in joint movement, the practitioner can better understand musculoskeletal conditions or injuries. Additionally, goniometers help evaluate treatment outcomes, document patient progress, and also detect issues early.

Using a Goniometer

A Goniometer consists of two arms connected by a pivot point and is typically made from clear plastic or metal.

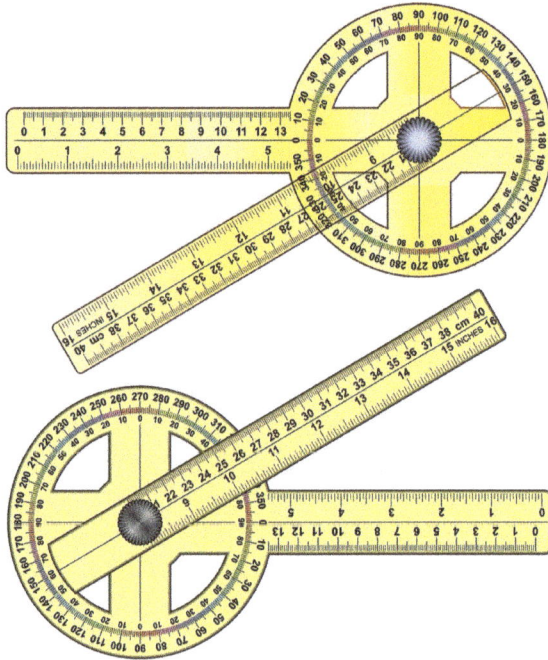

Goniometer

Before the examination, the patient is positioned comfortably, ensuring easy access to the assessed joint. The patient is informed about the process to ensure the patient understands what is being measured and is relaxed throughout the procedure.

To measure the range of motion, the practitioner accurately aligns the goniometer's pivot point with the joint's axis under evaluation. The axis represents the imaginary line around which the joint moves during its range of motion. For instance, in knee flexion and extension measurements, the goniometer's pivot point aligns with the knee joint's centre, and as the knee is flexed, the mobile arm of the goniometer is moved with the leg. The measurement on the goniometer dial is recorded. If the knee flexion angle is 120 degrees, this angle indicates the joint's range of motion in degrees, providing essential data for evaluation when compared to typical average range.

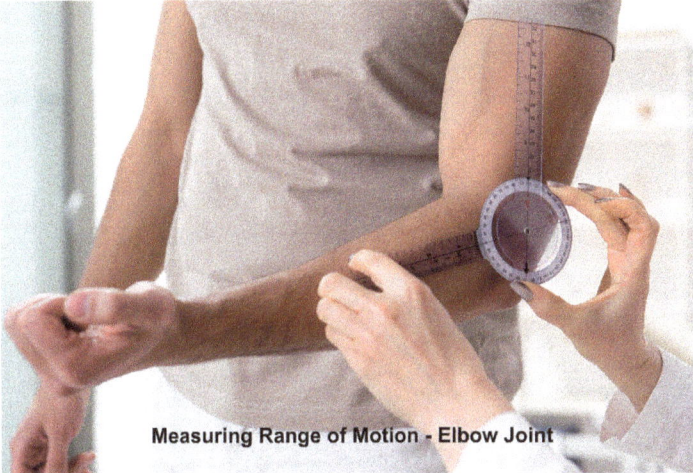

Elbow Joint ROM

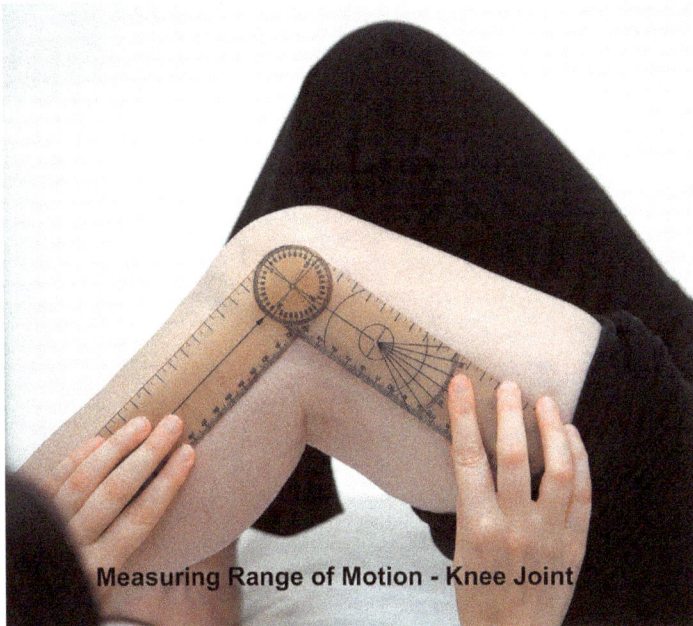

Knee Joint ROM

Joint	Position	Goniometer Placement	Movement	Measurement
Hip Flexion	Supine	Centre of axis of hip joint.	Raise knee towards chest.	Read flexion angle.
Hip Extension	Prone	Centre of axis of hip joint.	Move thigh backward.	Read extension angle.
Knee Flexion	Sitting or Supine	Centre of axis of knee joint.	Bend knee towards the buttocks.	Read flexion angle.
Knee Extension	Sitting or Supine	Centre of axis of knee joint.	Straighten knee.	Read extension angle.
Shoulder Flexion	Standing or seated	Centre of axis of shoulder joint.	Raise arm forward and upward.	Read flexion angle.
Shoulder Extension	Standing or seated	Centre of axis of shoulder joint.	Move arm backward and downward.	Read extension angle.
Elbow Flexion	Sitting or standing	Centre of axis of elbow joint.	Bend towards shoulder.	Read flexion angle.
Elbow Extension	Sitting or standing	Centre of axis of elbow joint.	Straighten forearm.	Read extension angle.

Table Showing Measurement Position of the Main Body Joints.

Conclusion

A comprehensive medical history guides the TCM practitioner to make informed decisions regarding diagnoses, treatment plans, and preventive measures. It also enables the practitioner to understand potential risk factors, anticipate complications, and identify interventions to suit the unique needs of each patient.

Chapter 11

Part 1 - Shoulder Anatomy

The shoulder joint, also known as the glenohumeral joint, is the main joint connecting the arm to the upper body. It is where the head of the humerus fits into a socket on the shoulder blade, the glenoid cavity. The shoulder joint is made up of a complex system of ligaments, tendons, and muscles, allowing for a wide range of movements. Ligaments provide stability by connecting bones to bones, while tendons connect muscles to bones. The surrounding muscles, including the rotator cuff muscles, play an important role in stabilizing and moving the shoulder joint. Due to its high degree of mobility, the shoulder joint is susceptible to various injuries and conditions, such as dislocations, rotator cuff tears, and arthritis.

Joints around the Shoulder

Glenohumeral Joint

The shoulder joint, or glenohumeral joint, is a complex ball-and-socket joint that connects the humerus to the scapula. It is one of the most mobile joints of the human body, allowing for a wide range of movements in multiple directions.[1] The range of motion which occurs at the shoulder includes is flexion, extension, abduction, adduction, external and internal rotation.

The normal range of motion at the joint is Flexion 180 degrees, Extension 45 – 60 degrees, Internal rotation 70 – 90 degrees, External rotation 90 degrees and Abduction 150 degrees.[2]

The shoulder joint is formed by the articulation of three bones:[3]

i) The humerus is the bone of the upper arm. It has a rounded head that forms the "ball" of the ball-and-socket joint. The head of the humerus articulates with the glenoid cavity of the scapula to form the shoulder joint.

ii) The scapula, also known as the shoulder blade, is a flat triangular bone on the upper back. It plays a vital role in the shoulder joint. The glenoid cavity, a shallow socket, is present on the lateral aspect of the scapula. It receives the head of the humerus, forming the ball-and-socket joint.

iii) The clavicle, commonly called the collarbone, is a long, S-shaped bone that connects the sternum to the acromion process of the scapula. Although the clavicle does not directly articulate with the shoulder joint, it provides structural support and helps maintain the shoulder complex's proper position.

Shoulder Joint Capsule

• The shoulder joint capsule, also known as the glenohumeral capsule, is a fibrous structure that surrounds the glenohumeral joint. The complex interaction between the fibrous layer, synovial membrane, ligaments, labrum, and other joint structures ensures the shoulder joint's stability and function.

• The outer layer of the shoulder joint capsule is composed of dense, fibrous connective tissue. This layer provides strength and structural integrity to the capsule. It consists of two parts, the fibrous capsule proper and the coracohumeral ligament. The fibrous capsule proper wraps around the joint and reinforces the joint's stability by connecting the humerus to the glenoid cavity of the scapula. The coracohumeral ligament which is an extension of the fibrous layer connects the coracoid process of the scapula to the greater tubercle of the humerus.

- The inner layer of the shoulder joint capsule is lined by a synovial membrane. The membrane covers the bones' articulating surfaces, lubricating the joint and secreting synovial fluid which provides nutrients to the joint.

- The labrum, a ring of fibrocartilage is attached to the outer edge of the glenoid cavity. Its function is to enhances the depth and provide stability to the joint by increasing the surface area for the humeral head to articulate within the glenoid cavity.

- The joint capsule contains nerve endings that provide sensory feedback about the joint's position, movement, and any potential changes. It also has blood vessels which supply nutrients and oxygen to the synovial membrane and other structures within the joint.

Sternoclavicular Joint (SC joint)

- The sternoclavicular joint situated at the front of the chest connects the medial end of the clavicle to the upper part of the sternum. Several ligaments provide stability to the sternoclavicular joint. The SC joint is the only bony connection between the upper limb and the axial skeleton transmitting forces from the upper limb to the trunk and allows a small degree of movement. The movements which take place include elevation and depression of the shoulder, as well as protraction and retraction of the clavicle. These movements allow for activities involving the arms and shoulders, such as lifting, pushing, and reaching. Injuries to the sternoclavicular joint are relatively rare but can occur due to severe trauma or dislocations.

Acromioclavicular Joint (AC joint)

- The acromioclavicular joint, is a small but crucial articulation located at the top of the shoulder. It is formed by the acromion, which is a bony process extending from the scapula, and the outer end of the clavicle. The joint is held together by strong ligaments and is enclosed by a capsule. Its function is to stabilize and facilitating movements of the shoulder complex. The AC joint is essential for various arm motions, particularly those involving raising the arm, rotating it, or carrying heavy loads.

The AC joint is prone to injuries, such as sprains, dislocations, or arthritis. These can occur due to trauma, repetitive stress, or degenerative changes over time.

Shoulder Ligaments

The glenohumeral joint has several ligaments which contribute to its stability and function to prevent excessive movement while allowing for a controlled range of motion. Injuries or problems with these ligaments can lead to shoulder instability, pain, and reduced functionality.

Some of the main ligaments found in the shoulder joint include:

- **Glenohumeral Ligaments:** This is a triad of ligaments; the superior glenohumeral ligament, middle glenohumeral ligament, and inferior glenohumeral ligament. These ligaments strengthen the joint's anterior aspect and prevent excessive forward movement of the humeral head. They also collectively strengthen the anterior aspect of the shoulder joint.

- **Coracohumeral Ligament:** Stretching from the scapula's coracoid process to the humerus's greater tubercle, the ligament contributes to stabilising the shoulder joint by restricting the downward movement of the humeral head. The ligament also assists in stabilising the joint during abduction and external shoulder rotation.

- **Coracoacromial Ligament**: A strong triangular ligament between the coracoid process and the acromion. The ligament is an integral component of the coracoacromial arch covering the shoulder joint, protecting the head of the humerus. The ligament *can* impinge and compress the rotator cuff muscle causing pain or discomfort. The tendon of the Coracoacromial ligament is prone to damage during a shoulder injury.

- **Transverse Humeral Ligament**: Also called Brodie's ligament, it forms a cover over the groove between the two tubercles of the humerus in the upper arm, holding the long head of the biceps tendon within this groove, preventing the biceps tendon from moving out of place The ligament acts as a pulley, maintaining the biceps tendon's position within the groove during arm movements.

- **The acromioclavicular ligament**: Connects the acromion process of the scapula to the outer end of the clavicle. Although not directly located within the shoulder joint, the acromioclavicular ligament has an important role in supporting the shoulder, preventing excessive upward movement of the clavicle, and upholding the correct shoulder alignment. Injuries to the acromioclavicular ligament, like strains or tears, can potentially induce shoulder instability, discomfort, and limitations in the shoulder joint's range of motion.

Shoulder Muscles

There are numerous muscles which surround and support the shoulder joint, enabling various movements of the upper arm, shoulder and the back. These muscles work together to provide stability, strength, and mobility to the shoulder complex.

The major shoulder muscles include:

Rotator Cuff Muscles: A group of four muscles surrounding the shoulder joint and playing a crucial role in its stability and movement. These muscles include:

- Supraspinatus: Originating from the supraspinous fossa of the scapula, it is responsible for initiating abduction (raising the arm to the side) and assists in maintaining the humeral head in the glenoid socket.

  Function - Initiates arm abduction.

- Infraspinatus: Originating from the infraspinous fossa of the scapula, it is involved in external rotation (rotating the arm outward) and provides stability to the shoulder joint.

  Function - External rotation

- Teres Minor: Originating from the lateral border of the scapula, it works in conjunction with the infraspinatus to aid in external rotation of the shoulder and provide stability.

  Function - assists in external rotation.

- Subscapularis: Originating from the subscapular fossa of the scapula, it is responsible for internal rotation (rotating the arm inward) and stabilisation of the shoulder joint.

  Function - Internal rotation.

The Deltoid: This is a large, triangular-shaped muscle that covers the shoulder joint. The muscle consists of three distinct parts:

- Anterior Deltoid: Originating from the front of the clavicle, it assists in shoulder flexion (lifting the arm forward and upward) and medial rotation (rotating the arm toward the body).

SHOULDER ANATOMY and ROTATOR CUFF MUSCLES

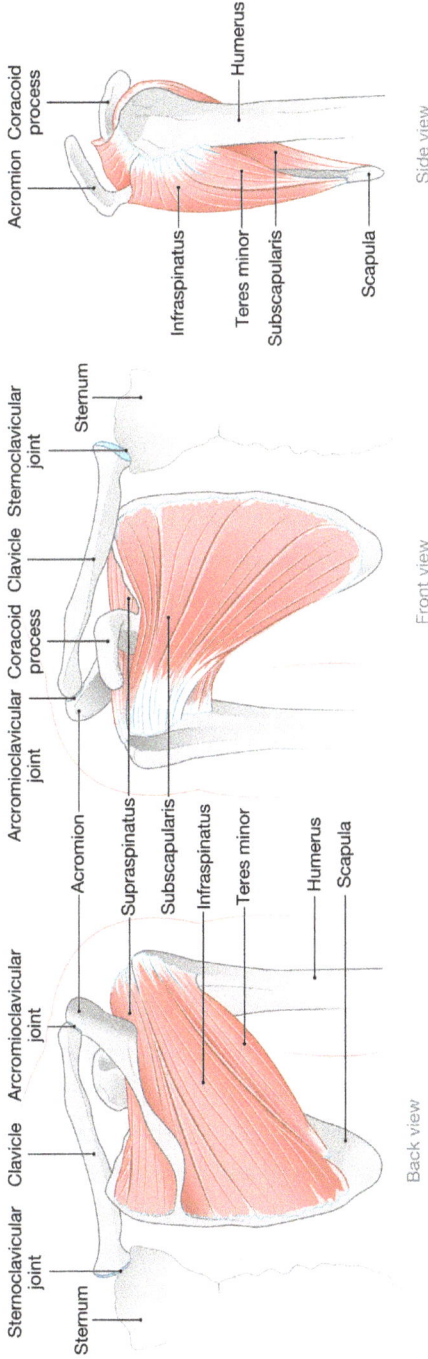

Back view

Front view

Side view

Shoulder anatomy Rotator Cuff

Sternoclavicular joint
Clavicle
Arcromioclavicular joint
Acromion
Supraspinatus
Subscapularis
Infraspinatus
Teres minor
Humerus
Scapula
Sternum

Arcromioclavicular joint
Coracoid process
Clavicle
Sternoclavicular joint
Sternum

Acromion
Coracoid process
Humerus
Infraspinatus
Teres minor
Subscapularis
Scapula

- Middle Deltoid: Originates from the acromion process of the scapula; it helps in shoulder abduction (raising the arm to the side) and is responsible for the initial elevation of the arm.

- Posterior Deltoid: Originating from the spine of the scapula, it contributes to shoulder extension (moving the arm backwards) and lateral rotation (rotating the arm away from the body).

Pectoralis Major: The pectoralis major is not naturally classified as a shoulder muscle, but it does play a significant role in shoulder movements due to its location and attachments. This large muscle is located in the chest, having two distinct heads:

- Clavicular (Upper) Head: Originating from the clavicle, it assists in shoulder flexion and horizontal adduction (bringing the arm across the body).

- Sternal (Lower) Head: Originating from the sternum, it contributes to shoulder extension and adduction.

Both the heads of the muscle attach to the clavicle, sternum, and ribs and insert onto the upper arm bone, the humerus.

Teres Major: While it is not directly classified as a shoulder muscle, it is closely associated with the shoulder complex due to its location and involvement in shoulder movements. Originating from the inferior angle of the scapula, it is situated below the infraspinatus. The teres major muscle works with the latissimus dorsi to aid shoulder adduction, extension, and medial rotation.

Biceps Brachii: While primarily known as a forearm muscle, the biceps brachii muscle has two heads originating from the scapula. The long head of the biceps crosses the shoulder joint and contributes to arm flexion, shoulder flexion, and supination (rotating the forearm to face upward).

Triceps Brachii: Located on the posterior aspect of the upper arm, the triceps brachii muscle has three heads (long head, lateral head, and medial head). While its primary function is elbow extension, it also contributes to shoulder extension.

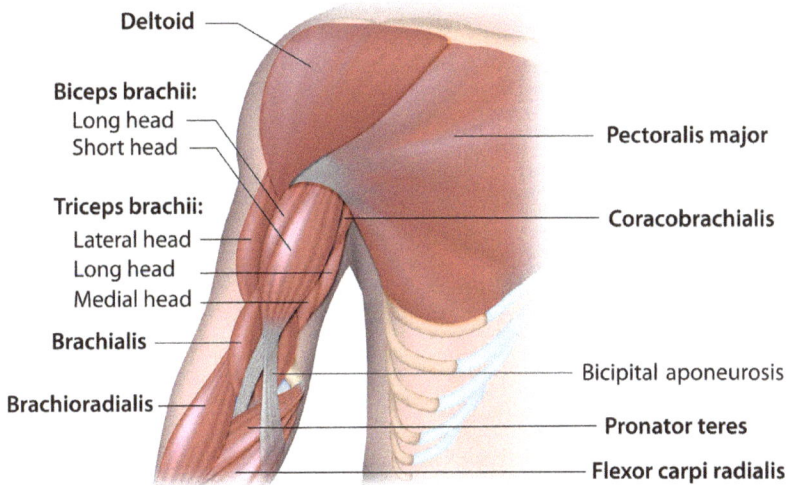

Deltoid

Biceps brachii:
Long head
Short head

Pectoralis major

Triceps brachii:
Lateral head
Long head
Medial head

Coracobrachialis

Brachialis

Bicipital aponeurosis

Brachioradialis

Pronator teres

Flexor carpi radialis

Shoulder Muscles

Latissimus Dorsi: often referred to as the "lats," is a large muscle located in the back, originating from the lower spine and iliac crest and inserts into the humerus. Its functions include arm extension, adduction and internal rotation. The latissimus dorsi also assists in various movements of the trunk and plays a role in maintaining overall back stability.

Trapezius: A flat, triangular muscle that covers the upper back and neck. It has three parts: upper, middle, and lower trapezius. The upper fibres elevate the scapula (shrugging the shoulders), the middle fibres retract the scapula (squeezing the shoulder blades together), and the lower fibres depress the scapula (lowering the shoulder blades). The trapezius is also involved in head and neck movements.

Serratus Anterior: Located along the sides of the ribcage, running from the upper ribs to the scapula. It plays a crucial role in protracting the scapula (moving it forward along the ribcage) and stabilizing the scapula during arm movements. This muscle is important for maintaining proper scapular positioning and allowing smooth overhead arm movements.

Levator Scapulae: The levator scapulae muscle runs along the side of the neck. It originates from the upper cervical vertebrae and inserts into the scapula. Its primary function is to elevate the scapula, assisting in shrugging the shoulders. The levator scapulae also contribute to head and neck movements and helps maintain the stability of the scapula.

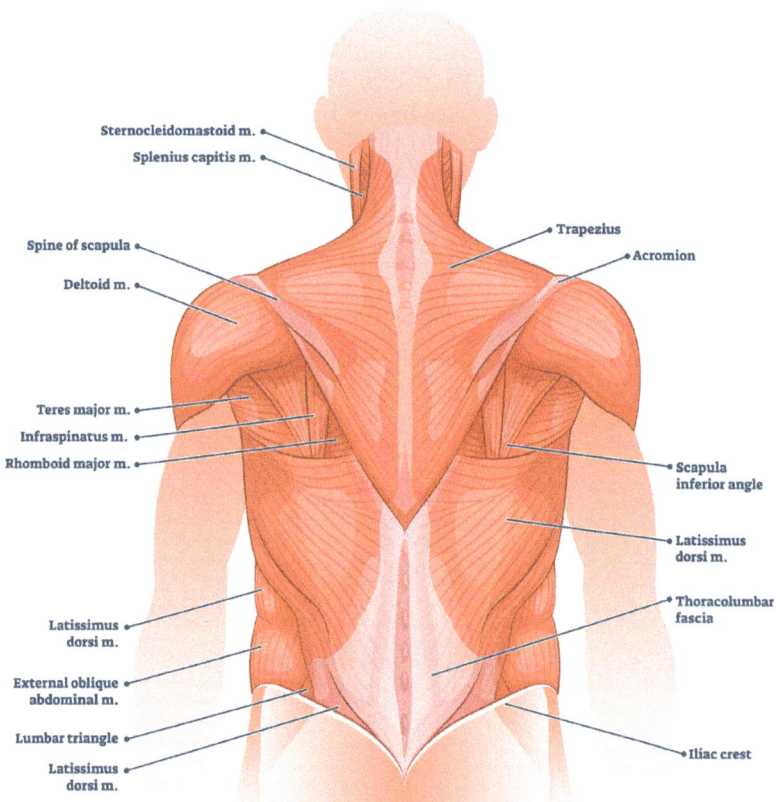

Back Muscles

Conclusion

The anatomy of the shoulder is well adapted to its function. The glenohumeral joint, acromioclavicular joint, and sternoclavicular joint collectively create a "joint system" that allows for a wide range of movements. The rotator cuff muscles are central in facilitating these movements and also for providing stability to the shoulder joint. Shoulder ligaments collectively maintain stability and provide structural support to the shoulder joint. The arrangement of the ligaments around the shoulder, whilst supporting movement also function to prevent injuries by stabilizing the shoulder joint. Due to its high mobility, the shoulder is also more prone to various injuries and conditions.

References

1. www: teachmeanatomy.info/upper-limb/joints/shoulder.
2. www.ncbi.nlm.nih.gov/books/NBK537018.
3. Levangie PK, et al. Joint Structure and Function. A comprehensive Analysis, 4th edition. JAYPEE 2006.

Chapter 11

Part 2 – Shoulder Injuries and TCM Treatment

As the shoulder joint is highly mobile and allows for a wide range of motion, this makes the shoulder susceptible to injuries, particularly in sports that involve repetitive overhead movements and throwing action. Due to this, shoulder injuries usually occur in sports such as baseball, swimming, tennis, volleyball, and weightlifting.[1] However, in sports, compared to other joints like the knee or ankle, shoulder injuries are not as prevalent as lower limb injuries.[2] When injuries do occur, this can have a significant impact on an athlete's performance and overall well-being.

Rotator cuff and Associated Injuries

The most common shoulder injuries in sports are injuries related to rotator cuff muscles.[3] Typically, injuries to these groups of muscles occur due to a combination of factors, including acute trauma or chronic wear and tear on the shoulder joint.

The causes of the injury include:

- **Acute Trauma**: Rotator cuff tears can result from a sudden, forceful injury to the shoulder. This can happen during sports activities, such as a fall onto an outstretched hand or a direct blow to the shoulder. Acute trauma can cause a partial or complete tear in the tendons of the rotator cuff.

- **Repetitive Movements**: Over time, repetitive overhead motions can lead to gradual wear and tear on the rotator cuff tendons, initially causing small tears to develop which may continue giving rise to complete tear of the muscles. This is common in athletes involved in sports like tennis, baseball, swimming, or weightlifting that require frequent and repetitive use of the shoulder joint.

- **Degenerative Changes**: With age, tendons of the rotator cuff muscles can undergo degenerative changes, becoming weaker and so more susceptible to injury. The blood supply to the tendons may decrease, reducing their ability to heal and so increasing the risk of tears. Factors like poor posture, improper lifting techniques, or inadequate shoulder conditioning can also accelerate degenerative changes.

Types of Rotator Cuff Injuries

Anatomically, the arrangement of the rotator cuff muscles within the shoulder joint allows for a high degree of motion but also exposes them to potential strain and friction. The joint's high mobility and load-bearing demands make the rotator cuff muscles essential for stability, yet the delicate balance between these factors can lead to wear and tear over time. Repetitive overhead movements common in activities like throwing, swimming, and weightlifting can overexert these muscles, causing microtrauma and inflammation. Also, age-related degenerative changes can weaken the tendons, and the limited blood supply to these tissues can slow down healing processes. Impingement and compression can further contribute to irritation and tears.

- **Rotator Cuff Tendinitis:** Rotator cuff tendinitis, also referred to as tendinopathy or tendonitis, is the inflammation or irritation of the rotator cuff tendons.

It commonly arises from overuse, repetitive motions, or degeneration of the tendons.

- **Impingement Syndrome:** Arises when the tendons of the rotator cuff get irritated and swollen while moving through the tight gap between the humerus and the acromion.

- **Partial Rotator Cuff Tears**: Partial tears occur when the rotator cuff tendon sustains damage but remains partially intact without complete severance. They can develop due to repetitive stress, sudden trauma, or a combination of factors.

- **Full-Thickness Rotator Cuff Tears**: Full-thickness tears are more severe than partial tears, also known as complete tears, and involve a complete severance or detachment of the rotator cuff tendon from the bone. They can be caused by acute traumatic events like heavy falls or forceful movements and chronic degeneration over time.

- **Calcific Tendinitis:** In this condition, calcium deposits form in the tendons of the rotator cuff, leading to pain and limited movement. It can be associated with chronic inflammation.

Sports associated with rotator cuff injuries include tennis, swimming, volleyball, basketball, gymnasts, badminton and weight lifters, and most sports with overhead action.

General Symptoms of Rotator Cuff Injuries:
- Pain which can radiate down the arm. Pain at night, especially when lying on the affected shoulder.

- Weakness of the shoulder and difficulty in activities that require lifting, pushing, or pulling.

- Reduced range of motion in the shoulder.

- Some patients with rotator cuff injuries might feel a sense of shoulder instability or "looseness."

- Rotator cuff injuries can cause clicking, popping, or grinding sensations when moving the shoulder.

- Certain movements or actions can exacerbate the pain associated with a rotator cuff injury, for example, activities like reaching overhead, throwing, lifting heavy objects.

- If a rotator cuff injury is severe or long-standing, it can lead to muscle atrophy in the affected area.

- Patients with rotator cuff injuries can experience pain and discomfort when trying to sleep on the affected shoulder.

- Tenderness to touch around the injured area and localized swelling can be present due to inflammation and irritation of the damaged tendon.

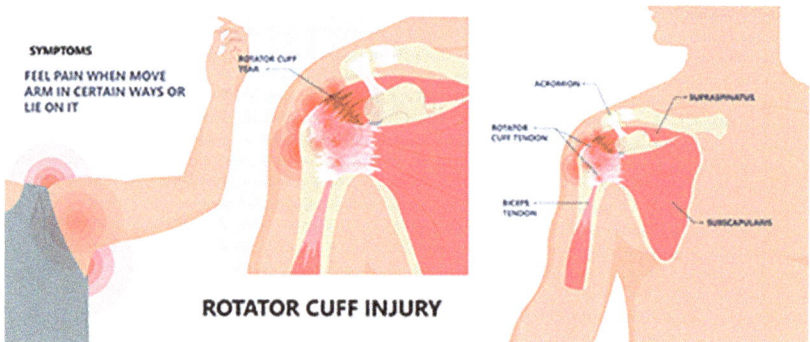

Rotator Cuff Injury

Impingement Syndrome

Shoulder impingement syndrome occurs when the structures within the subacromial space, located between the humerus and the acromion, experience compression or pinching. This narrow space contains the rotator cuff tendons, the long head of the biceps tendon, and the subacromial bursa. Compression or pinching of the tendons, bursa, or biceps tendon within the subacromial space leads to inflammation and irritation, resulting in shoulder impingement syndrome. This condition manifests as pain, weakness, and limited range of motion, especially during activities that involve overhead movements. Several factors can contribute to the compression, including structural abnormalities like a curved or hooked acromion, weakness or imbalances in the rotator cuff muscles, overuse or repetitive overhead movements, and poor posture. Shoulder impingement can coexist with other shoulder conditions, such as rotator cuff tears or biceps tendonitis, which can further worsen symptoms and complications.

Common Symptoms of Shoulder Impingement:

- The "painful arc": In shoulder impingement, this refers to a specific range of motion in which the patient experiences pain or discomfort. It typically occurs during the middle phase of raising the arm from a resting position at the side of the body to an elevated position above shoulder level. Identifying the painful arc is an important diagnostic indicator.

- Discomfort and pain: This is the primary manifestation of shoulder impingement, often localized in the front or side of the shoulder and occasionally extending down the arm.

- Discomfort during arm movement: Pain intensifies when elevating the arm, particularly when lifting it to the side or extending it overhead.

- Muscle weakness: Some patients may experience diminished strength in the affected arm, especially when engaging in activities requiring lifting or exertion.

- Difficulties with overhead asks: Tasks like retrieving items from high places, grooming activities, or putting on clothing may become more demanding and painful.

- Restricted range of motion: There may be limitations in freely moving the arm, particularly in actions involving arm elevation or rotation.

- Audible clicking or popping sensation: Some patients may perceive a clicking or popping sensation in the shoulder when moving the arm.

- Tenderness to touch: Sensitivity to touch may be present over the *front or side* of the shoulder, where impingement occurs.

- Night-time discomfort: In certain instances, individuals with shoulder impingement may experience heightened discomfort at night, particularly when lying on the affected side.

- Muscular tightness: The muscles surrounding the shoulder may become tense or rigid, adding to the discomfort.

Symptoms of shoulder impingement usually develop gradually over time, often starting mildly before becoming more pronounced.

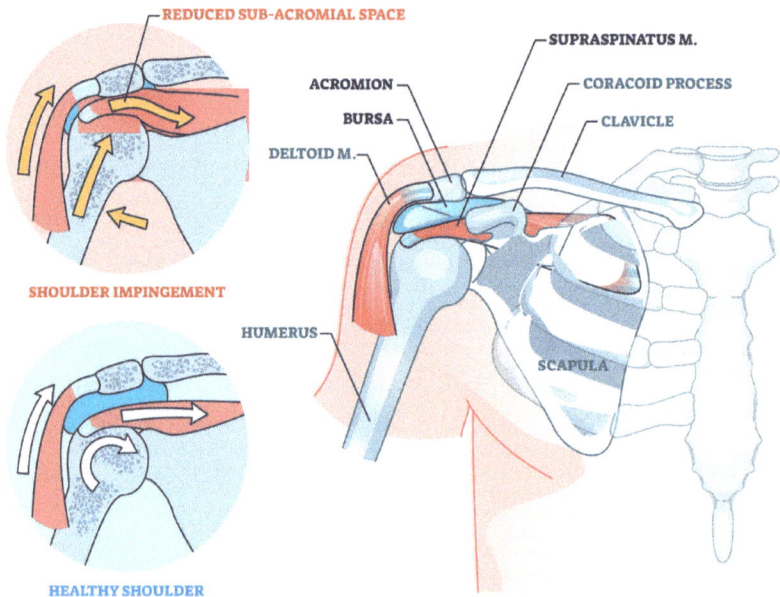

Shoulder impingement

Characteristic	Shoulder Impingement	Rotator Cuff Injuries
Cause	Compression and irritation of tendons/ bursa between acromion and humeral head.	Damage to rotator cuff muscles/ tendons (inflammation, tears).
Pain	Outer part of shoulder, radiates down arm, aggravated by overhead movements.	Localized deep shoulder pain, may radiate down arm.
Painful Arc	Present; pain during arm elevation (60-120 degrees).	Not a defining characteristic.
Weakness	Possible weakness in arm lifting.	Weakness specific to affected muscle.
Range of Motion	Limited range of motion, especially in overhead tasks.	Decreased range of motion, based on affected muscle.
Pain at rest	Generally, less likely; pain often tied to movement.	Possible pain at rest, especially during sleep.
Specific Weakness	Not necessarily tied to specific muscle.	Specific muscle weakness based on affected muscle.
Symptoms	Pain with specific movements, difficulty reaching behind back, clicking/snapping.	Pain, weakness, functional limitations, muscle atrophy.

Differences Between Rotator Cuff Injuries and Shoulder Impingement.

Biceps Tendinopathy

Biceps tendonitis is an inflammatory condition that primarily affects the long head of the biceps tendon, which extends through the front of the shoulder joint and attaches to the top of the glenoid socket. It is typically caused by repetitive overhead movements like throwing a baseball, serving in tennis, or performing weightlifting exercises such as bicep curls or overhead presses.

Repetitive stress on the biceps tendon can lead to microtrauma, inflammation, and irritation, resulting in tendonitis. Biceps tendonitis may also be linked to other shoulder conditions like rotator cuff tears or shoulder impingement.

Symptoms of Biceps Tendinopathy Include:

- Pain in the front of the shoulder: A common symptom is persistent, deep-seated pain in the front of the shoulder. It may worsen with certain movements, particularly overhead activities or when lifting heavy objects.

- Pain radiating down the arm: The pain may radiate along the front of the upper arm, sometimes extending down to the elbow. This can occur particularly during activities that involve bending or straightening the arm.

- Tenderness over the Biceps groove: The area where the biceps tendon passes through the bicipital groove may be tender to touch.

- Weakness in arm strength: Some individuals with biceps tendinopathy may experience weakness in activities that require forceful use of the arm, such as lifting or carrying.

- Pain with specific movements: Pain may be triggered by specific movements, such as reaching overhead, lifting heavy objects, or resisting against resistance.

- Clicking or popping sensation: Some individuals may experience a clicking or popping sensation in the shoulder, particularly when moving the arm.

- Difficulty with rotational movements: Movements that involve rotating the forearm, such as gripping a racquet or even turning a key, may exacerbate the pain.

- Worsening pain at night: In some cases, patients may experience an increase in pain during the night, particularly if they sleep on the affected side or in a position that puts pressure on the shoulder.

- Stiffness and reduced range of motion: Over time, biceps tendinopathy can lead to stiffness and limited range of motion in the affected shoulder.

Labrum Strains and Tears

The labrum, a fibrous structure that lines the rim of the glenoid and provides additional support to the joint can be subjected to various types of injuries, including strains, tears, and other damage.

The labrum can experience excessive stress or tension, leading to microtears or inflammation in the tissue. This can happen due to repetitive movements, overuse, or sudden trauma. Sports that involve overhead motions or forceful throwing, such as baseball or tennis, can put significant strain on the labrum.

Symptoms of a strained labrum include shoulder pain, a sensation of catching or popping in the joint during movement, decreased range of motion, and potentially weakness. As the labrum continues to be stressed and if microtears remain they can progress into larger tears. These tears can be partial, involving a portion of the labrum, or complete, where the entire labrum is torn away from the

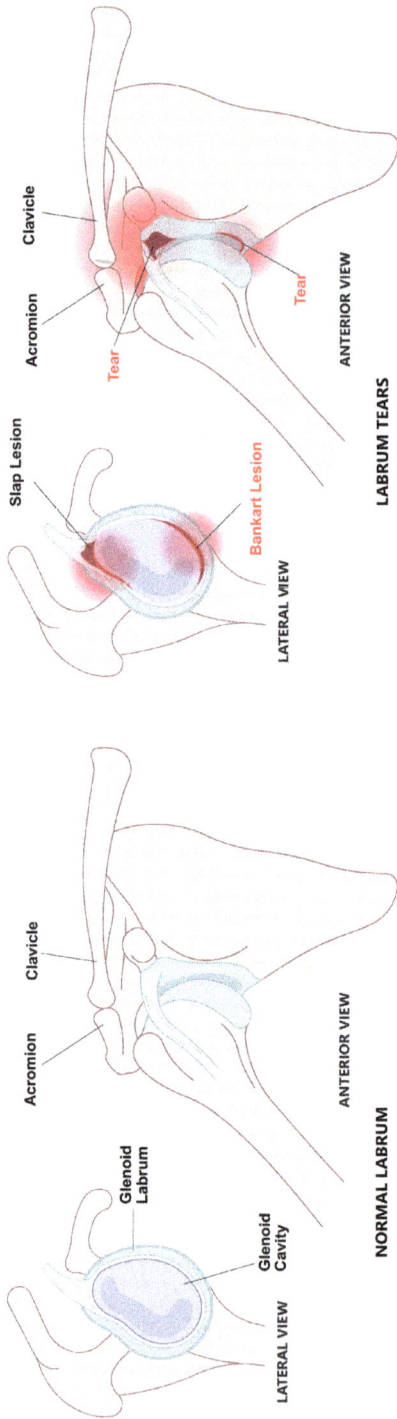

Shoulder labrum tears

LABRUM TEARS

Clavicle

Acromion

Tear

Tear

ANTERIOR VIEW

Slap Lesion

Bankart Lesion

LATERAL VIEW

NORMAL LABRUM

Acromion

Clavicle

ANTERIOR VIEW

Glenoid Labrum

Glenoid Cavity

LATERAL VIEW

glenoid socket. As the tear progresses, symptoms can become more pronounced with increased pain, a sensation of catching or popping in the shoulder joint, decreased range of motion, and potential weakness. The shoulder might also feel less stable.

TCM Treatment of Shoulder Injuries

Shoulder injuries in sports often stem from direct impact during contact sports, leading to fractures, dislocations, or soft tissue damage. Moreover, repetitive overhead movements like throwing or swimming can cause conditions such as rotator cuff tears, tendonitis, or bursitis. Incorrect form or technique in activities like weightlifting, tennis, or golf can strain the shoulder joint and surrounding muscles. Weaknesses or imbalances in these muscles may also contribute to instability and vulnerability to injury. Specific injuries like rotator cuff tears, labral tears, or shoulder dislocations can occur due to sudden movements or repeated stress.

In TCM, the concept of pathology involves imbalances in the flow of Qi and Blood within the body's meridians, as well as disruptions in the balance between Yin and Yang, presenting with various syndrome patterns. While the specific conditions of rotator cuff injuries, shoulder impingement, biceps tendinopathy and labral tears have distinct modern medical explanations and treatments, TCM looks at these conditions as imbalances. Acupuncture points are selected based on their ability to restore harmony to these imbalances.

Local and Adjacent Points

Please see Appendix 1 for Acupuncture Point Location.

Using local and adjacent acupuncture points during an acute injury is contradicted as inserting needles into inflamed, swollen tissues might worsen the injury, cause more pain, or increase inflammation. Additionally, there's a risk of bleeding or infection, particularly if the skin is compromised. The discomfort of acupuncture could add to the existing pain, and also its pain-relieving effects might mask the injury's severity, potentially delaying necessary medical attention. However, using acupuncture in subacute injuries is beneficial, focusing on a combination of local and adjacent points to optimize the body's healing response, improve blood flow, alleviate residual discomfort, and promote tissue repair without directly aggravating the still-recovering injury site.

Large Intestine Meridian Points

- **LI15:** *The primary point for shoulder disorders.* Also called the "energy vortex" point for the shoulder, it benefits the shoulder and alleviates pain, regulates Qi and Blood, clears heat, dispels wind-damp and dredges connecting vessel. Useful point for rotator cuff tendonitis, shoulder impingement (similar to LI16), motor impairment of upper extremities, and bursitis.

  Needling: 1.0cun to 1.5cun, perpendicular towards the centre of the axilla (avoid deep needling as the apex of the lung can rise 2 – 4cm).

  Useful in early subacute injuries, when there is redness, heat and muscle spasm with the inability to raise the arm above shoulder level. Combine with LI12 and SI4.

  Also useful in early subacute injury with redness, swelling and heat sensation, especially when LI15 is combined with LI14. The point is also useful when the shoulder has a painful obstruction, particularly Wind-Damp.

  LI15 can be combined with LU5, SI8, PC7, SI3 and LU10 if the elbow is also affected.

- **LI16:** Although mainly for chronic injuries, LI16 can be used in the subacute phase of the injury. It clears Blood

Stasis, alleviates pain and benefits the shoulder. Combine with LI15.

Needling: 0.5cun to 1.0cun oblique, perpendicular (caution deep needling can cause pneumothorax).

- **LI14:** Used when pain radiates from shoulder to elbow or upwards from elbow to shoulder, frozen shoulder and neck rigidity. Also, supporting point for LI15.

Needling 1cun to 1.5cun, perpendicular or oblique (that is, horizontal and upwards)

Some points below, on the Small Intestine Channel, can be beneficial for shoulder and scapular pain, but can carry a substantial risk of pneumothorax. When using these useful points, the practitioner **must** *have anatomical knowledge of the lung/chest area. The athlete's build will also guide the depth of needling. It may be useful to be aware of the following symptoms of pneumothorax;*

- *Sudden Chest Pain, often felt on the side of the collapsed lung which is exacerbated by breathing or coughing.*

- *Shortness of Breath*

- *Tachypnoea (Rapid Breathing)*

- *Cyanosis*

- *Persistent cough*

- *Decreased Chest Movement*

- *Subcutaneous Emphysema – causing a crackling sensation or sound when touched.*

When needling any points which carry a risk of pneumothorax, the patient must be informed of the above symptoms as sometimes the condition may develop immediately but also later after treatment.

Small Intestine Meridian Points

- **SI9:** Used for pain and stiffness around the scapular region and when pain radiates to the upper thoracic region (T1 to T6) and upper arm. Activates the channel and alleviates pain. SI9 also expels Wind and benefits the shoulder (Bi Syndrome).

  Needling: 1cun to 1.5cun, perpendicular.

- **SI10** is useful for injuries in the early subacute phase when shoulder muscles are in spasm. If used during this phase of the injury, combine with ST38 (needled first) and SJ14, LI15 and SI6. SI10 can also be used as a substitute for SI9. SI10 is frequently used for shoulder injuries; it is a meeting point for three channels that pass through the shoulder; Small Intestine, Yang Linking, and Yang Motility.

  Needling: 1cun to 1.5cun, perpendicular.

- **SI11** is used when pain is felt in the scapular region and when pain radiates to the lateral posterior aspect of the elbow. SI11 is a valuable point for rotator cuff pathologies and frozen shoulder when the athlete finds it painful to raise or rotate the arm. Combine with SI4 when the arm is involved and is painful.

  Needling: 0.5cun to 1cun, perpendicular or oblique

- **SI12** or **SI13** as they have similar properties as SI11, but using either of these points (SI12 or SI13) also benefits the sinews and reduces pain, so are useful in shoulder tendinopathy, especially for the rotator cuff group of muscles. Caution: Needling these points carries a **substantial pneumothorax** risk, so needling must be precise.

- Needling SI12: 0.5cun to 0.8cun (so not quite cun !), using oblique medial insertion, directed towards the spine.

  Needling SI13: 0.5cun to 0.8cun, oblique lateral insertion.

If the scapular area is also painful, combine with SI11 and SI9.

- **SJ13** clears the channels and invigorates the collaterals, benefitting the shoulder and alleviating pain. It also clears the channel and regulates Qi. Point is useful when shoulder pain also radiates to the upper arm.

  Needling: perpendicular, 1.0cun to 1.5cun, directed towards the axilla.

- **SJ14** benefits the shoulder by invigorating Qi and Blood, relieving pain. A good point to use for rotator cuff pathologies, such as shoulder impingement and tendinopathy, especially if the symptoms are on the lateral aspect. SJ14 is beneficial for frozen shoulder when combined with ST38. When using this combination, ST 38 is needled first, and the patient is asked to rotate the shoulder whilst manipulating the needle (caution as muscle can be in spasm, this can result in a "stuck needle" effect). Combine with LI14, SJ5 and LI4.

  Needling: perpendicular, 1.0cun to 1.5cun, directed towards the axilla.

- **SJ15** has a similar action to SJ14 but is useful to use when pain extends to the elbow, or there is neck stiffness. Needling this point carries a substantial risk of **pneumothorax**, especially if needled perpendicular and deep.

  Needling: 0.5cun to 0.8cun, oblique insertion, the direction of which depends on the presenting symptoms.

Additional Points

- **GB21** is used when pain may be at the top of the shoulder area (near the acromioclavicular joint) with stiffness and rigidity along the neck (combine with BL42). Point is also useful if the pain is present in the upper back thoracic region (up to T 7) when it can be combined with BL12, SJ3 and SJ6 and BL40.

Although beneficial for the above symptoms, using this point carries a substantial risk of pneumothorax if needled incorrectly or needled deep. Use of this point is contraindicated in pregnancy and if the patient has a history of cardiac complaints.

Needling: Always needle posterior 0.5cun to 0.8cun, although some texts also recommend a perpendicular insertion.

- If there is pathology of the acromioclavicular joint (as mentioned earlier), use points LI11 or LI10 with LI4 and ST37. You can also use a combination of LI15 and LI16.

- **Extra local point:** Jianqian/Jianneiling is located midway between the acromioclavicular joint and anterior axillary fold. Vertical insertion, up to 1.5cun. Opens the channel and Luo connecting vessel locally.

- **LI4** combined with **Liv3 - four gates:** Circulate Qi and Blood and helps to open all the meridians, increase circulation, and so decrease pain anywhere in the body

Distal Points

Distal points, which are below the knees and elbows are chosen as they open the channel to eliminate stagnation of Qi and so Blood. When used during the early subacute phase, use the reducing method. For post-acute and chronic injuries, use the even method.

When choosing distal for treating shoulder injuries, the meridian affected is identified as this determines the choice of acupuncture points. For example, if the pain is along the anterior aspect of the shoulder, choose points along the Lung channel; if the pain is along the lateral aspect, then points along the Large Intestine Channel are chosen.

The meridians around the shoulder are:

- Small Intestine Channel on the posterior aspect.
- Lung and Pericardium Channels on the anterior aspect.
- Large Intestine Channel on the Lateral aspect.
- San Jiao Channel on the lateral aspect.
- Gall Bladder Channel on top of the shoulder

Distal points act to open the channel by eliminating the stagnation of Qi. In Bi Syndrome, distal points also expel pathogens within the body (see below). The rule of thumb is that distal points are chosen from the channel affected by the injury. However, this need only sometimes be the case, as distal points from one channel can affect another channel. Distal points are needled first as this will clear the obstruction in the channels and open the channels, facilitating the use of local and adjacent points later in the treatment.

Distal points for shoulder injuries

- **Stomach channel - ST38.** This is the empirical point for all painful shoulder disorders, frozen shoulder and shoulder tendinopathy. Expels wind-damp activates meridian, alleviates pain and benefits the shoulder.

  Needling: Perpendicular 0.5cun to 1cun. Needle on the affected side, whilst the athlete rotates the shoulder around the area of pain. Combine with local shoulder points as described above.

- **San Jiao Channel - SJ5** is an important distal point for channel disorder affecting the shoulder with referral symptoms affecting the arm, elbow and wrist. SJ5 activates the channel, alleviates pain, expels wind (Wind–Heat), and releases the exterior—a useful point for scapular pain.

Needling: Perpendicular 1.0cun to 1.5cun. Caution, after insertion (as the needled area is between the radius and ulna), if the patient moves the arm during treatment, this could bend the needle (depending on the individual's bony structure).

- **Small Intestine Channel - SI3** relaxes sinews on the SI channel. Activates channel and alleviates pain at scapula (combined with SI4, BL12 and GB21), stiff neck (combined with SJ16) and elbow pain.

  Needling: Perpendicular 0.5cun to 1.0cun

- **Large Intestine Channel - LI4** Influences circulation of Qi and Blood, activates channel and alleviates pain, strengthens Wei Qi and calms the spirit. Used for pain anywhere in the body when it is combined with Liv3 (four gates)

  Needling: Perpendicular: 0.5cun – 1.0cun. It is contraindicated in pregnancy.

- Also, use **GB34** to relax and strengthen sinews and bones. Removes obstruction from channels so Qi and Blood flow to alleviate pain and stiffness. It can be used for sinews and joint problems all over the body (not just the shoulder).

  Needling: Perpendicular 1cun to 1.5cun. Needle the affected side.

- **SJ10** is used as it activates the channel and alleviates pain when the shoulder, elbow, arm, neck as well upper lumbar is afflicted with painful obstruction syndrome.

  Needling: Perpendicular: 0.5cun – 1.0cun.

Corresponding Points for Shoulder

For pain relief, and in acute conditions when local and adjacent points are not chosen, corresponding points can be used. These points will be shoulder/hip points. The corresponding point will be identified by finding painful points at the injury site and then using the appropriate corresponding point on the hip.

PC2 to LIV2, LU2 to SP12, LI15 to ST30, SJ14 to GB30 and SI10 to BL39

Auricular Points

Shen Men: Found near the apex of the triangular fossa of the antitragus, this point is considered a master point for pain and stress relief. It can help alleviate overall tension and discomfort.

Point Zero: This central point in the ear is often used for overall pain management and can have a balancing effect on various bodily systems.

Shoulder Point (AH SHI or Shoulder 1): This point is located at the superior border of the scapula on the ear. It's one of the primary points targeted for shoulder pain and dysfunction.

Upper Limb Point (Shoulder 2): Found just below the Shoulder Point, this point corresponds to the upper limb and can be useful for treating pain and discomfort in the shoulder area.

Subcortex (A Hunger Point): This point is located at the apex of the triangular fossa of the antihelix. It's often used for pain management and can be beneficial for various types of pain, including shoulder pain.

Clavicle (Shoulder 3): This point is situated near the upper border of the antitragus, at the junction of the ear's helix and antihelix. It's used to target the clavicle and shoulder area.

Scapula (Shoulder 4): Located adjacent to the Superior Antihelix Crus, this point corresponds to the scapula and can be targeted for shoulder issues.

Sympathetic Autonomic Point: Located in the area where the antihelix meets the helix, this point is targeted for general pain relief and relaxation.

Endocrine Point: Situated near the centre of the ear, this point corresponds to the endocrine system and can be used to address hormonal imbalances that might contribute to pain and inflammation.

Adhesive Capsulitis

Adhesive capsulitis, or frozen shoulder, is not typically a common sports injury and so is considered separately. While it can occur in individuals who participate in sports activities, it is not directly caused by sports-related trauma or acute injuries. However, prolonged periods of arm immobilisation, such as after surgery or injury, can increase the risk. Adhesive capsulitis more commonly develops due to other factors, such as inflammation, thickening, and tightening of the shoulder capsule over time. These factors can be associated with conditions like shoulder impingement, rotator cuff tears, or underlying medical conditions like diabetes or thyroid disorders, so it may interest TCM practitioners.

The exact cause of adhesive capsulitis is not fully understood, but it is believed to involve an abnormal inflammatory response and scar tissue formation within the capsule. This process leads to a progressive loss of both active and passive shoulder mobility. Adhesive capsulitis is characterised by inflammation, thickening, and tightening of the shoulder joint capsule. The shoulder capsule is a tough connective tissue structure that surrounds and stabilises the joint while allowing for a wide range of motion.

Adhesive capsulitis typically develops in three distinct stages, Freezing, Frozen and the Thawing stage. The symptoms associated with the three stages and the acupuncture points are:

Freezing Phase

- Gradual emergence of shoulder pain, often felt deep within the joint. This pain might be more acute at night or when lying on the affected side.

- Growing discomfort and stiffness with shoulder movements. Everyday actions that involve reaching, lifting, or moving the arm away from the body can become increasingly difficult.

- The range of motion of the shoulder starts to decline, particularly in terms of external rotation (outward arm turning) and abduction (lifting the arm sideways).

Acupuncture Points

- **LI15:** Located on the upper arm, LI15 can help alleviate shoulder pain and stiffness.

- **SI10:** Found on the upper arm, SI10 eases shoulder pain and improve range of motion.

- **LU2:** This point on the upper chest can help with pain and discomfort in the shoulder area.

Frozen Phase

- Although the pain may reduce compared to the freezing phase, it can persist, especially during movements that stretch the shoulder capsule.

- Stiffness remains a prominent issue, making routine activities a challenge.

- The ability to move the shoulder becomes considerably restricted. Basic tasks like dressing, reaching, or grooming can be quite difficult.

Acupuncture Points

- **LI16:** Located on the shoulder, LI16 can provide relief from ongoing stiffness and discomfort.

- **TB15:** Situated on the upper arm, TB15 is used to address shoulder pain and limited range of motion.

- **GB21:** Located on the shoulder, GB21 is a commonly used point for various shoulder issues, including frozen shoulder.

Thawing Phase

- Pain typically subsides significantly during this phase, although discomfort may still arise during specific movements or activities.

- Stiffness gradually lessens, and movements become more comfortable.

- The range of motion in the shoulder starts to recover, facilitating enhanced flexibility and smoother daily tasks.

Acupuncture Points

- **LI4:** Found on the hand, LI4 can help improve overall circulation and relieve pain.

- **GB34:** Situated on the lower leg, GB34 can help with pain management and enhance the flow of Qi.

- **ST38:** This point on the lower leg is sometimes used to improve blood circulation and alleviate pain.

- **SP10:** Located on the thigh, SP 10 can be useful for addressing pain and discomfort.

Bi Syndrome of the Shoulder

When Bi syndrome affects the shoulder, it is typically called "Bi Zheng" of the shoulder and refers to a syndrome characterized by obstruction and stagnation in the channels and collaterals, often resulting in pain, stiffness, and limited range of motion in the affected area.

The aetiology of Bi syndrome can be multifactorial, including external pathogenic factors (such as Wind, Cold, Dampness, and Heat), as well as internal factors like Qi and Blood stagnation, deficiency, or a combination of these.

For Bi syndrome of the shoulder, points are selected which correspond to the affected meridians and focus on moving Qi and Blood, relieving pain, and promoting circulation.

Acupuncture points for shoulder Bi syndrome include:

GB21: Located on the highest point of the shoulder muscle, GB21 is frequently used for shoulder pain and stiffness.

LI15: Found on the lateral side of the upper arm, LI15 is used to alleviate shoulder pain and improve range of motion.

TE14: Located on the posterior aspect of the shoulder, TE14 is another important point for shoulder pain and immobility.

SI9: Situated on the posterior shoulder and often used for shoulder pain and stiffness.

LU7: Although located on the wrist, LU7 can be used for Bi conditions affecting the shoulder.

LI4: Located on the hand, LI4 is a versatile point used for various pain conditions, including those involving the shoulder.

SJ14: Located on the scapula, SJ14 is used for shoulder and scapular pain.

Ashi points: These are tender points found along the affected area. Needling these points can help relieve pain and tension.

Conclusion

Rotator cuff and associated anatomical structure injuries, can be a common source of shoulder pain and dysfunction, affecting athletes. These injuries can result from trauma, overuse, or degeneration, leading to symptoms such as pain, weakness, limited range of motion, and difficulty performing daily activities. While conventional treatments like physical therapy, medication, and surgery can be effective, Traditional Chinese Medicine offers a holistic and complementary approach to managing rotator cuff injuries.

TCM views health as a balance between the body's Qi and the harmony of its systems. By inserting fine needles into specific acupuncture points, practitioners aim to restore the flow of Qi, reduce inflammation, and promote the body's natural healing processes. Points along meridians associated with the shoulder, such as those linked to the Large Intestine and Small Intestine, can be targeted to alleviate pain and improve range of motion. Additionally, points associated with overall wellbeing, like Lung and Spleen points, may be used to address any underlying imbalances contributing to the injury.

References

1. M. Oberlander, A. Chisar, and B. Campbell, "Epidemiology of shoulder injuries in throwing and overhead athletes," Sports Medicine and Arthroscopy Review, vol. 8, 2000.
2. Clin J Sport Med. 2010 Jul;20(4):256-63.
3. HB Park, SK Lin, A Yokota, Clinics in sports, sportsmedtheclinics.com

Chapter 12

Part 1 – Elbow Anatomy

The elbow joint is a synovial joint connecting the humerus to the two bones of the forearm, the ulna and the radius. The elbow joint allows for the flexion and extension of the forearm and some rotational movements. It is primarily classified as a hinge joint due to its ability to perform bending and straightening actions, similar to the hinge of a door. However, it also has some pivot joint characteristics, allowing for pronation (inward rotation) and supination (outward rotation) of the forearm. The range of motion at the elbow is 130-155 degrees of flexion, 5 degrees of extension (unless hyper-extended), pronation approximately 75-85 degrees and supination 80–105 degrees.[1]

The elbow joint is uniquely adapted to meet the demands of sports activities. These adaptive features of the elbow joint allow athletes to perform a wide range of motions, generate power, maintain stability, and protect against injury while engaging in sports activities. In throwing and pitching sports, like baseball, softball, and cricket, the elbow joint provides necessary extension and flexion movements for generating power and accuracy during throwing motions. With racquet sports, such as tennis, badminton, and squash, the elbow joint's structure is designed to generate powerful shots, and the joint facilitates the extension and flexion required to swing the racquet and transfer energy to the ball. The elbow joint also provides a supporting role. For example, in golf, although the elbow joint is not directly involved in the swing motion, it helps to maintain proper arm and wrist alignment, contributing to a smooth and controlled swing. Incorrect swing mechanics or overuse can lead to conditions like golfers' elbow, which involves inflammation of the tendons on the inner side of the elbow.

Structure of the Elbow Joint

The upper arm bone, the humerus, connects to the two bones of the forearm, the ulna and the radius. The humerus has two bony prominences known as the medial and lateral epicondyles, which are attachment points for muscles and ligaments.[2] The ulna is one of the two bones of the forearm and is located on the arm's medial aspect (inner side). It forms the more significant part of the elbow joint and has a bony projection called the olecranon process, which forms the bony tip of the elbow. The radius is the other forearm bone on the arm's lateral aspect (outer side). It is shorter and thinner than the ulna and plays a role in the elbow joint by allowing for rotational movements of the forearm.

The elbow's joint capsule comprises an outer fibrous layer and an inner synovial layer. It provides stability, protection, and lubrication to the elbow joint, enabling smooth and controlled movement.

Ligaments of the Elbow Joint

The function of ligaments at the elbow joint is to provide stability by connecting bones together. They help to hold the bones in proper alignment and prevent excessive movement or dislocation of the joint during various activities. Ligaments, listed below also play an important role in protecting the joint from injuries or excessive stress

Medial Collateral Ligament (MCL), also known as the Ulnar Collateral Ligament, has three components;

- The anterior bundle runs from the humerus's medial epicondyle to the ulna's tubercle, serving as the primary stabilizer against valgus stress (see below).

- The posterior bundle, located behind the anterior bundle, adds extra stability against valgus stress by extending from the medial epicondyle to the proximal part of the ulna.

- The Transverse Ligament, a thinner and more superficial part of the MCL, connects the anterior and posterior bundles, further enhancing stability on the inner side of the elbow joint.

Lateral Collateral Ligament (LCL) or Radial Collateral Ligament originates from the lateral epicondyle of the humerus. It attaches to the annular ligament and the lateral side of the radius bone. The LCL provides stability to the outer aspect of the elbow joint and resists varus stress (see below).

Annular Ligament is a strong and circular band that encircles the head of the radius bone, keeping it in place against the ulna. It enables smooth rotation of the radius during pronation and supination movements of the forearm.

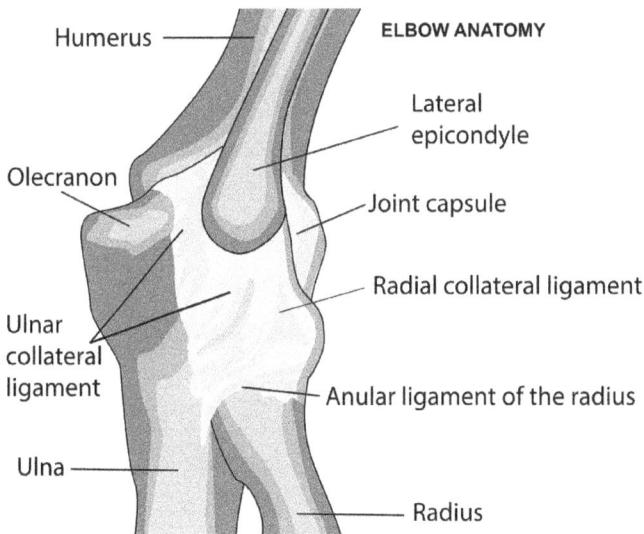

ELBOW ANATOMY

Humerus

Lateral epicondyle

Olecranon

Joint capsule

Radial collateral ligament

Ulnar collateral ligament

Anular ligament of the radius

Ulna

Radius

Elbow anatomy

Interosseous Membrane is not an actual ligament. It is a fibrous sheet which connects the radius and ulna bones along their lengths. It promotes stability in the forearm and assists in distributing forces between the two bones during different movements.

Valgus Stress

When the arm is bent at the elbow, and an external force pushes the hand in a direction away from the body, this is known as valgus stress. When the elbow has excessive valgus stress it can lead to various potential outcomes.[3] One common result is the strain or potential tearing of the ulnar collateral ligament (located on the medial side). Apart from ligament-related issues, excessive valgus stress can compromise joint stability, potentially increasing feelings of looseness, increased joint mobility, and a greater susceptibility to partial dislocation or dislocation. Prolonged exposure to valgus stress might trigger chronic inflammation and irritation due to the repeated strain on the UCL and adjacent structures, potentially leading to conditions like "golfer's elbow" and other injuries resulting from overuse.

Varus Stress

Varus stress, which is the opposite of valgus stress, in the elbow joint, involves an inward or sideways force applied to the outer part of the joint. This force results in the joint opening or widening on the inner side. Varus stress commonly arises when an external force pushes the joint inward or towards the body's midline.[4]

Muscles acting on the Elbow Joint

Several muscles, below, work together to provide stability and movement at the elbow joint.

- **Biceps Brachii:** The biceps brachii is a two-headed muscle on the anterior or front of the upper arm. It originates from the shoulder girdle and attaches to the radius bone in the forearm. The biceps brachii functions as a powerful flexor of the elbow joint, allowing for movements such as lifting and curling the arm. The biceps brachii muscle is involved in various sports movements, particularly in activities like weightlifting, throwing, and striking in baseball, boxing, and tennis. The biceps brachii also assists in shoulder flexion and forearm supination. The primary function is elbow flexion.

- **Triceps Brachii:** The triceps brachii is a three-headed muscle located on the posterior or back of the upper arm. It originates from the shoulder girdle and the scapula attaching to the ulna bone in the forearm. The triceps brachii is the primary extensor of the elbow joint, enabling movements like straightening the arm. Triceps brachii also plays a role in sports like weightlifting, throwing, and striking, where powerful arm extension is required. The triceps brachii is particularly active in overhead presses, push-ups, javelin throwing, and volleyball spikes.

- **Brachialis:** The brachialis is a muscle situated underneath the biceps brachii. It originates from the front of the humerus and attaches to the ulna bone in the forearm. The brachialis acts as a powerful elbow flexor, working alongside the biceps brachii to flex the elbow joint. It is an essential muscle for sports activities involving powerful arm flexions, such as weightlifting, grappling, and combat sports like boxing and mixed martial arts.

- **Brachioradialis:** The brachioradialis muscle is located on the outer side of the forearm. It spans from the upper arm to the radius bone. The brachioradialis is involved in forearm flexion and is particularly active during actions such as lifting or pulling. While it does not directly act on the elbow joint, it assists in activities like curling and hammering movements. The brachioradialis is active in sports such as golf, baseball (bat swings), and racquet sports like tennis and badminton.

- **Pronator Teres:** The pronator teres is a muscle on the forearm's inner side. It originates from the humerus and

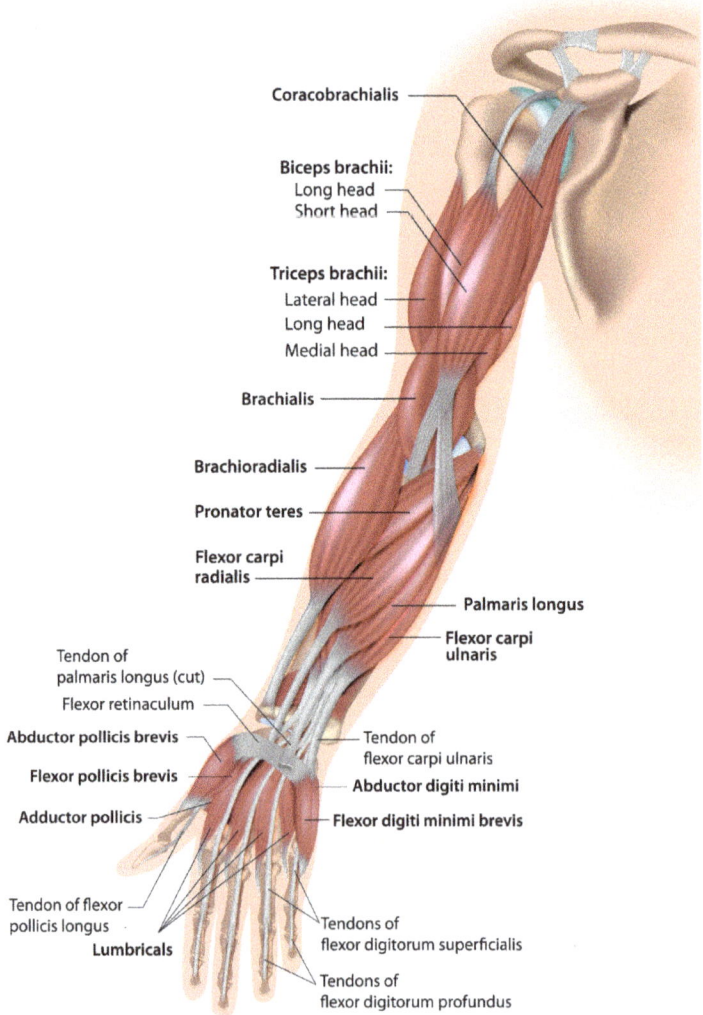

Muscles of the arm

attaches to the radius bone. The pronator teres plays a role in pronation, which involves rotating the palm of the hand downward. The pronator teres and other forearm muscles provide the necessary rotational force and control during sports activities requiring forearm pronation. It plays a vital role in achieving accuracy, power, and control in various sports movements and contributes to overall performance involving rotational actions of the forearm.

- **Anconeus muscle:** This is a relatively small and triangular muscle. It lies deep in the triceps brachii muscle and is visible as a distinct muscle near the elbow joint. The anconeus muscle is located on the posterior aspect of the forearm, specifically on the lateral aspect. It originates from the lateral epicondyle of the humerus and attaches to the posterior surface of the ulna bone in the forearm.

Conclusion

The elbow's anatomy plays an important role in supporting various movements and actions. The elbow joint, formed by the humerus, radius, and ulna, acts as a synovial joint that enables the controlled extension, flexion, and rotation of the forearm.

However, the dynamic and demanding nature of sports can subject the elbow to significant stresses and forces, leading to a range of injuries. Ligaments, tendons, and muscles surrounding the elbow are prone to strain, sprain, or overuse. Medial and lateral collateral ligaments, essential for stability, can become vulnerable during forceful motions or sudden impacts. Additionally, conditions such as tennis and golfer's elbow highlight the intricate interplay between muscles, tendons, and joints.

References

1. www.ncbi.nlm.nih.gov/PMC6555111
2. Kerkhof FD, van Leeuwen T, Vereecke EE. The digital human forearm and hand. J Anat. 2018 Nov.
3. Hotchkiss RN, Weiland AJ. Valgus stability of the elbow. J *Orthop Res.* 1987;
4. Magee, D. J. (2014). Orthopedic Physical Assessment-E-Book. Elsevier Health Sciences.

Chapter 12

Part 2 – Elbow Injuries and TCM Treatment

The elbow in its central position of the upper body kinetic enables athletes to carry out a diverse range of movements, from powerful throws to delicate manoeuvres. However, the very complexity that gives the athletes the ability to carry out these activities also exposes the elbow to a spectrum of potential injuries.

Lateral Epicondylopathy (Tennis Elbow)

* Lateral epicondylopathy, also known as tennis elbow, is a painful condition that involves the inflammation or degeneration of the tendons that attach to the lateral epicondyle of the humerus. This condition is characterized by pain and tenderness on the outer part of the elbow, which can sometimes radiate down the forearm. The primary cause of lateral epicondylopathy is repetitive overuse and strain on the extensor tendons and muscles that attach to the lateral epicondyle, which is the bony prominence on the outer side of the elbow. This overuse leads to microtears, inflammation, and degeneration of the tendons over time causing pain, inflammation, and discomfort in the outer part of the elbow.

The main anatomical structures affected include:

* The tendon most frequently affected in tennis elbow is the Extensor carpi radialis brevis (ECRB) tendon.

The ECRB muscle and its associated tendon function in extending the wrist which enables the upward movement of the hand. Repeated stress on this tendon, resulting from actions like gripping and recurrent wrist extensions, can cause tiny tears, inflammation, and deterioration.

- The tendons of several forearm muscles come together to form a common extensor tendon that attaches to the lateral epicondyle of the humerus.[1] These tendons collectively contribute to wrist and finger extension. As with the ECRB tendon, the common extensor tendon is also affected primarily due to repetitive strain and overuse, leading to microtears, inflammation, and degeneration.

- Radial collateral ligament which helps stabilize the elbow joint, can become irritated and inflamed which can contribute to the pain experienced in tennis elbow.

- The Annular ligament which surrounds the radial head, helps to stabilize the elbow joint. While not a primary site of damage in tennis elbow, it can be indirectly affected due to its proximity to the inflamed area.

Causes of Lateral Epicondylopathy:

- Engaging in sports that involve repetitive gripping, lifting, or swinging motions can strain the tendons that attach to the lateral epicondyle. Sports like tennis, golf, and weightlifting often require these repetitive actions, which can lead to overuse and strain on the tendons.

- Using incorrect techniques while playing sports can place excessive stress on the forearm tendons.

- Sports that involve forceful impacts or collisions, such as contact sports like football or rugby, can lead to sudden strains on the tendons and contribute to the development of lateral epicondylopathy.

- Using sports equipment, such as tennis rackets or golf clubs, with improper grip sizes or that are not suited to the athlete's hand size and strength can increase the risk of developing tennis elbow.

- Athletes who participate in intense training sessions without allowing adequate time for recovery may be at higher risk.

- Failing to properly warm up the muscles and tendons before engaging in sports can increase the likelihood of strain and injury, including lateral epicondylopathy.

- Imbalances in the muscles and mechanics of the upper extremities can alter the distribution of forces during sports activities, leading to increased strain on the lateral epicondyle.[3]

- Rapidly increasing the intensity or duration of sports activities without gradual progression and conditioning can strain the tendons and contribute to the development of tennis elbow.

- Age-related changes in the tendons, such as decreased flexibility and increased susceptibility to degeneration, can increase the risk of developing lateral epicondylopathy in older athletes.

Symptoms of Lateral Epicondylopathy:

- The most common symptom is pain, on the outer part of the elbow, specifically around the bony prominence, the lateral epicondyle. The pain is sharp, burning, or aching in nature. It often starts mildly and gradually worsens over time as the injury progresses.

- There is tenderness to touch over the lateral epicondyle, and sometimes this tenderness can extend along the forearm muscles.

- Activities that involve gripping, lifting, and repetitive wrist extension, such as shaking hands, turning a doorknob, lifting objects, or using tools, can trigger or exacerbate the pain.

- There may also be weakness in the grip strength due to discomfort and pain felt when using the hand and wrist.

- Stiffness in the elbow joint and forearm muscles may be present, especially after periods of rest.

- The pain might radiate down the forearm, affecting the muscles and tendons that are involved in wrist and finger movements.

Test for Lateral Epicondylopathy

A simple test called the Cozen's Test can be carried out to diagnose tennis elbow. This involves asking the patient to extend their wrist against resistance, which can reproduce pain if the condition is present.

Golfers Elbow (Medial Epicondylopathy)

- Medial epicondylopathy, also termed golfer's elbow or thrower's elbow, primarily arises due to the repeated strain and overuse of the forearm muscles and tendons connected to the inner elbow's bony prominence, the medial epicondyle.

The main anatomical structures affected include:

- Medial epicondylopathy, or golfer's elbow, primarily affects the muscles and tendons located on the inner side of the forearm which attach to the medial epicondyle of the humerus bone in the upper arm. The muscles most commonly affected include pronator teres, flexor carpi radialis and flexor carpi ulnaris. These muscles collectively play a role in wrist and hand movements involved in gripping, lifting, and performing activities that require wrist flexion and forearm pronation. When these muscles are repetitively strained or subjected to overuse, they can develop small tears, leading to inflammation and pain around the medial epicondyle.

Causes of Medial Epicondylopathy:

- Repetitive strain is the main cause of medial epicondylopathy induced by repetitive movements, causing small tears in tendons due to the recurring stress.[2] This process leads to inflammation and resultant pain.

- Activities like golf (hence the term "golfer's elbow") and throwing in sports like baseball and tennis where there a strong grip and repetitive wrist flexion contributes to this condition.

- Using incorrect techniques during sports or tasks intensifies strain on the forearm tendons, heightening the risk of injury.

- Abruptly starting a new activity or escalating an existing one without appropriate conditioning strains the tendons, contributes the onset of medial epicondylopathy.

- As age advances, tendon flexibility can naturally decrease, making tendons more susceptible to injury. Age-related degenerative changes in tendons increases the risk of developing medial epicondylopathy.

Symptoms of Medial Epicondylopathy:

- Pain is the classic symptom of medial epicondylopathy. The pain is experienced on the inner side of the elbow, in close proximity to the medial epicondyle. This pain can manifest as a localized sensation or radiate along the forearm. Activities that involve actions like gripping objects, lifting items, or flexing the wrist, or even performing routine wrist movements, tend to exacerbate the pain.

- Athletes affected by medial epicondylopathy feel a sense of diminished strength and weakness in the arm that is experiencing the condition. This weakness can impede tasks that require a strong grip or involve flexion of the wrist, making activities like carrying heavy objects or engaging in sports more challenging.

- Stiffness can be a secondary symptom, particularly noticeable after periods of rest or upon waking in the morning. The elbow joint and the forearm may feel rigid and less mobile.

- The area around the medial epicondyle can become tender and sensitive to touch. Pressing on or near this region can elicit discomfort.

- Accompanying the condition, sensations of numbness or tingling that travel from the inner side of the elbow down the forearm may be felt. These sensations could indicate potential involvement of nerves passing through the affected area.

- Engaging in activities requiring forceful gripping, wrist flexion, or repetitive wrist movements can intensify the discomfort. Actions like executing motions involved in golf swings or racket sports can trigger or worsen the symptoms.

- Other symptoms may include neck stiffness and median nerve irritation.

Some texts may refer to lateral and medial epicondylitis. Although these terms may still be used, they are not strictly correct, as the "itis" suggests inflammation. Inflammation is only present in the earliest stage of the disease, whereas the chronic stages are more attributable to a degenerative process.[4] Using the term medial epicondylopathy for the golfer's elbow and lateral epicondylopathy for the tennis elbow is the preferred terminology.

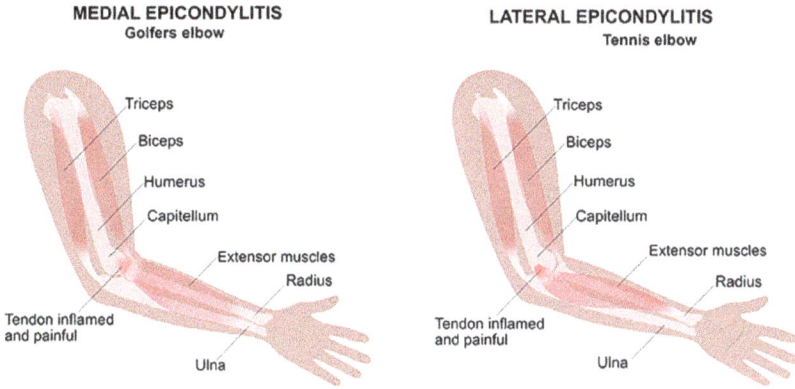

Epicondylitis

Elbow Sprains

Elbow sprains occur when the ligaments surrounding the elbow joint are stretched or torn due to excessive force or sudden, awkward movements. The structures primarily affected are the ligaments around the elbow joint. The main ligaments involved in elbow stability are:

- Medial Collateral Ligament.
- Ulnar Collateral Ligament.
- Lateral Collateral Ligament.
- Annular Ligament.

Causes of elbow sprains include:

- Direct Trauma: A sudden impact or blow to the elbow can stretch or tear the ligaments.
- Forceful Twisting or Rotation: Sudden twisting or rotation of the forearm, especially when the arm is extended, can lead to sprains.

- Hyperextension: Bending the elbow beyond its normal range of motion, such as during a fall, can strain or tear the ligaments.

- Overuse or Repetitive Stress: Athletes who engage in repetitive motions that stress the elbow, such as throwing or serving in tennis, can develop chronic sprains over time.

The severity of an elbow sprain can range from mild (stretching of the ligaments) to severe (complete tear of the ligaments).

Elbow Strains

Elbow strains, also known as muscle strains or pulls, occur when the muscles or tendons around the elbow are stretched or torn due to excessive force or overuse.[3] This can happen in various sports or activities that involve repetitive or sudden movements of the forearm and elbow.

Muscles Affected:

- Flexor Muscles: These muscles are located on the anterior aspect of the forearm and are responsible for flexing the elbow. The primary flexor muscle in this region is the biceps brachii, which also helps in flexing the shoulder.

- Extensor Muscles: These muscles are located on the posterior side of the forearm and are responsible for extending the elbow. The main extensor muscles include the triceps brachii.

- Forearm Supinator and Pronator Muscles: These muscles are responsible for rotating the forearm. The supinator turns the palm upward, while the pronator teres and pronator quadratus muscles turn the palm downward.

Causes of Elbow Strains:

- Overexertion or Overuse: Engaging in repetitive motions or activities that strain the muscles and tendons around the elbow, such as repetitive throwing or swinging in sports like baseball, tennis, or golf, can lead to strains.

- Sudden Forceful Movements: A sudden, forceful movement of the forearm or elbow, such as a quick and abrupt change in direction, can strain the muscles and tendons.

- Improper Technique: Using incorrect or poor technique in sports or activities can place excessive stress on the muscles and tendons around the elbow, increasing the risk of strain.

- Lifting Heavy Objects: Lifting heavy objects, especially with improper form, can strain the muscles and tendons around the elbow.

- Falls or Trauma: Falling onto an outstretched arm or experiencing a direct impact to the elbow can result in strains.

The symptoms of an elbow sprain and strain can be quite similar, as both injuries involve damage to the soft tissues around the elbow joint. Common symptoms shared by both elbow sprains and strains include;

- Pain is a primary symptom in both elbow sprains and strains. It may be localized around the elbow joint and can range from mild to severe.

- The affected area can be tender to the touch, indicating inflammation or injury to the soft tissues.

- Both injuries can lead to swelling around the elbow, due to the body's natural response to tissue damage.

- Reduced range of motion may be experienced, making it difficult to fully extend or flex the elbow.

- The affected arm may feel weaker than usual, especially when using the muscles involved in the injury.

- Depending on the severity of the injury, bruising (discoloration of the skin) may develop around the elbow.

- Some patients may experience a popping or snapping sensation at the time of injury, which can be indicative of a strained or sprained ligament or muscle.

- In more severe cases, there may be associated nerve compression or irritation, leading to sensations of numbness or tingling radiating down the arm.

- Certain movements or activities, such as lifting objects, gripping, or extending the arm, may exacerbate the pain.

- While the symptoms are similar, it is important to note that an elbow sprain specifically refers to an injury to the ligaments around the joint, whereas an elbow strain relates to an injury of the muscles and tendons.

Summary of Other Injuries Which Occur at the Elbow

- **Olecranon bursitis** which is a fluid-filled sac located at the tip of the elbow, can become inflamed due to repeated pressure or trauma. This can result in a swollen, painful, and sometimes tender bump at the back of the elbow.

- **Ulnar nerve compression** or Cubital Tunnel Syndrome which is compression or irritation of the ulnar nerve as it passes through the cubital tunnel can lead to symptoms such as numbness, tingling, and weakness in the forearm and hand. Repetitive bending of the elbow can exacerbate this condition.

- **Radial tunnel syndrome** is similar to nerve compression. Radial tunnel syndrome involves the compression of the radial nerve, resulting in pain and discomfort on the outer side of the elbow and forearm.

- **Avulsion injuries** involve the tearing away of ligaments or tendons from their attachment points on bones. They can occur due to sudden forceful movements or collisions.

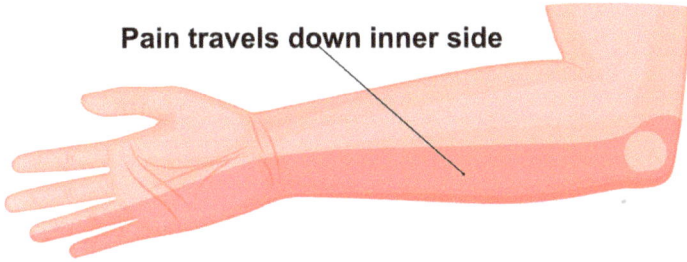

Pain travels down inner side

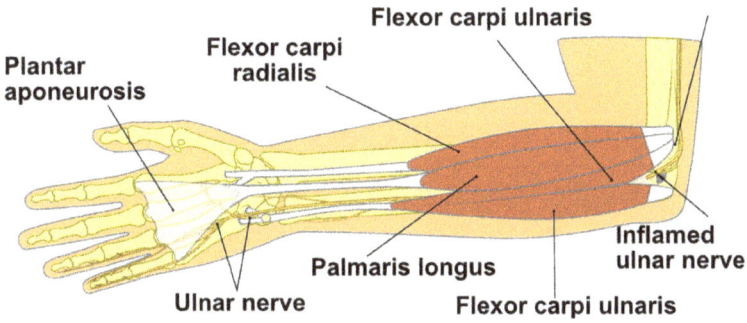

Plantar aponeurosis

Flexor carpi radialis

Flexor carpi ulnaris

Palmaris longus

Ulnar nerve

Inflamed ulnar nerve

Flexor carpi ulnaris

Cubital Tunnel pain Syndrome

Elbow injuries, whether caused from sudden impacts, repetitive motions, or inadequate technique, demonstrate the delicate balance between the elbow's versatility and vulnerability. From strains and sprains to overuse conditions, these injuries can disrupt an athlete's performance and overall well-being.

TCM Treatment of Elbow Injuries

The injuries above, such as medial and lateral epicondylopathy, and elbow sprains have been explained in Western Medical terminology. Although this description can help the TCM practitioner better understand the nature of the injury, in TCM the above injuries are seen as irregularities in the circulation of Qi and Blood Stagnation along the body's meridians and as imbalances in the equilibrium between Yin and Yang. These irregularities manifest through various syndrome patterns. TCM interprets these conditions as disruptions in balance for which acupuncture points are chosen based on their potential to reinstate harmony to these imbalances.

During the subacute phase which follows an acute stage, and which can last for several weeks after the initial injury local, adjacent, distal and Ashi points can be used, depending on the injury's severity and the presenting symptoms. If swelling and other signs of acute inflammation are still present at the site of the injury or condition, needling local points is not advised as this may cause a further inflammatory response including pain and so exacerbate the inflammatory response. Instead, adjacent and distal points can be used. During acute phase, PRICE – protection, rest, ice, compression and elevation is used.

Local and Adjacent points for Elbow Injuries

Please see Appendix 1 for Acupuncture Point Location.

- **LI11:** A useful point to use in the early stages of inflammation of tennis elbow or golfers' elbow as it cools pathogenic Heat (both internal and exterior), activates channels to regulate Qi and Blood, alleviates pain, and nourishes the tendons. The point also "opens" the elbow joint and so will reduce stiffness. It can act as a distal point if the shoulder is also symptomatic. LI11 is also useful in eliminating the exterior.

  LI11 can be combined with GB21 or LI10 and SI3 (when the forearm is also symptomatic).

Needling: Perpendicular, 1.0cun to 1.5cun with elbow flexed

- **LI10:** Point on the Yangming channel, which is abundant in Qi and Blood. Using this point invigorates the circulation of Qi and Blood in the elbow and the upper arm. As LI10 is a beneficial point in chronic elbow injuries, the temptation is to use it frequently. Over-needling of this point can be avoided by alternating using LI11 (and LI10). Both these points can also be combined. It also dispels Wind.

  When there is difficulty in flexing and extending the arm (pain and stiffness around the elbow and forearm), combine LI10 with LI6. When the elbow has chronic pain, use ST36 to "boost" Qi and Blood and improve circulation.

  Needling: Perpendicular, 1.0cun to 1.5cun

- **LI12:** Benefits the elbow joint, so it is the primary local point used for elbow symptoms, mainly when pain is also referred to the shoulder. If the condition is acute with redness and swelling, combine with LI15 and SI4. LI12 can also be used as a substitute point if LI11 cannot be used or when LI10 has been over needled.

  Needling: Perpendicular 0.5cun – 1.0cun

- **PC3:** Activates channel and alleviates pain. Clears Heat and Cools Blood and so indicated for conditions associated with Heat and inflammation. PC3 also reduces local swelling and inflammation.

  Needling: Perpendicular insertion, approx. 0.5 to 1cun. Caution while needling as brachial artery and vein lie medial to the point.

- **LU5:** This is another valuable point to use as it occupies a central position on the Lung Channel, so it affects the whole upper limb, mainly when flexion and extension are limited. It can be used for wandering pain (Wind and

Wind-Damp) with elbow and shoulder stiffness. If LI11 is ineffective, use LU5 as it is a local point which should be directed towards the area of stagnation, especially if the injury is tennis elbow. It can be combined with GB38, which relaxes the sinews, activates the channel and alleviates pain. Another valuable combination for elbow pain and stiffness is LU5 and LI11. LU5 also relaxes the sinews.

Needling: Perpendicular 0.5cun to 1.0cun

- **SJ10:** Useful point in the early stages of an elbow injury for tendonitis (inflammation) as it clears Heat from the channel and activates it, thus alleviating pain. SJ10 is useful for Bi Syndrome and also when pain is referred to the arm, shoulder and neck.

  Needling: Perpendicular 0.5cun to 1.0cun.

- **SI8:** As SI8 removes obstruction from the channel, this is an excellent point to use when symptoms are around the small intestine channel. It can also be used to treat shoulder, forearm, and shoulder disorders. It also clears Heat and Damp-Heat.

  Needling: Perpendicular, with the elbow flexed, 0.3cun – 0.5cun *Caution: very sensitive point to needle; warn patient!*

Distal Points and Meridians

These points below the elbow and knees open the channels to eliminate Qi and Blood Stagnation and treat pathologies proximal to the distal points. Distal points act to open the channel by eliminating the stagnation of Qi. In Bi Syndrome, distal points also expel pathogens within the body (see below). The rule of thumb is that distal points are chosen from the meridian affected by the injury. However, bear in mind that distal points from one channel can affect another channel.

Distal points are used first to clear the obstruction in the channels and also to open the channels, facilitating the use of local and adjacent points later in the treatment.

On the anterior aspect the meridians around the elbow are:

- Large Intestine Meridian of Hand Yangming: The Lung meridian follows a pathway along the radial side of the forearm and extends from the hand to the chest region.

- Pericardium Meridian of Hand Jueyin: While this meridian doesn't directly pass through the elbow, it is connected to the arm and is associated with the heart's protective functions. It influences emotions and the circulation of Qi and Blood.

- Heart Meridian of Hand Shaoyin: The Heart meridian passes along the ulnar side of the forearm and is related to heart health, emotions, and the circulation of Blood and Qi.

On the posterior aspect the meridians around the elbow are:

- Small Intestine Meridian of Hand Taiyang: This meridian runs along the ulnar side of the arm and passes through the elbow. It starts from the outer tip of the little finger and travels up the arm. It is associated with the Small Intestine organ and its related functions.

- Triple Burner Meridian of Hand Shaoyang: This meridian is not directly connected to the elbow but has branches that run through the forearm. It is associated with regulating the body's fluid metabolism and Qi distribution.

- The Large Intestine Meridian of Hand Yangming: Does not directly pass through the elbow joint, instead it runs along the arm on the radial side, starting at the index finger and extending up the arm, crossing the wrist, and continuing further along the forearm.

- Liver Meridian of Foot Jueyin: While not directly related to the elbow, the Liver meridian has branches that affect the forearm. It's associated with the Liver organ's functions related to detoxification, emotions, and the smooth flow of Qi.

Distal Points

- **ST35:** (or ST36) is used here as the upper/lower point, YangMing's corresponding point. ST36 is preferred if the pain is more symptomatic in the extensor group and ST35 when pain is around the lateral epicondyle.

   The side to use is determined by the stage of the injury: The opposite side when acute and the same side when chronic.

   Needling: 0.5cun to 1.0cun with knee slightly flexed, needling 1cun to 1.5cun

- **LI4:** Influences and promotes the smooth flow of Qi and Blood in the whole arm. It also activates channels and alleviates pain, strengthens Wei Qi and calms the spirit. The primary point to expel Wind-Cold, Wind-Heat and to release the exterior.

   Needling: Perpendicular: 0.5cun – 1.0cun. Caution do not use in pregnancy.

- **SJ4:** Useful point when the wrist is also affected as part of the kinetic chain. Relaxes sinews and alleviates pain.

   Needling: slightly oblique and proximal, towards the elbow, 0.3cun to 0.5cun. Sensitive point to needle, warn the patient.

- **SJ5:** Important confluent point of the Yang linking channel, linking the six Yang and Governing channels. *For properties, see the section below on Bi Syndrome.*

Needling: Slight oblique towards the ulnar side, 0.5cun to 1.5cun. Caution when needling, movement by the patient's arm can result in a "bent needle."

- **GB34**: Main point for soothing, relaxing and strengthening sinews and joints (as related to the Liver) eliminates stagnation, Wind Damp and activates channel and alleviates pain.

  Needling: Perpendicular 1cun to 1.5cun. Needle the affected side.

- **LI14**: Positioned on the upper arm, around the midpoint between the shoulder and elbow. Activates the channel and alleviates pain. LI14 can be effective for addressing pain and discomfort in the elbow and upper arm area. If difficulty raising arm, use in combination with LI12.

  Needling: Oblique insertion, up to 1.5cun

Elbow and Knee Corresponding Points

For elbow injuries or other musculoskeletal conditions, corresponding points are typically used when the primary acupuncture meridians that pass through the elbow (such as the Large Intestine, Small Intestine, and Triple Burner meridians) may not provide sufficient relief on their own. Corresponding points allow TCM practitioners to directly target the affected area, facilitating healing and pain relief. It is important to note that while corresponding points can be effective in treating elbow injuries, they are often used in conjunction with points along the primary meridians associated with the affected area. Additionally, the specific points chosen will depend on the individual's unique condition, diagnosis, and the practitioner's assessment.

HT3 to KID10, PC3 to LR8, LU5 to SP9, LI11 to ST35, SJ10 to GB34 and SI8 to BL40

Auricular Points

- Elbow Point: This point is located on the upper part of the earlobe, near the border of the helix. It corresponds to the elbow area and can be used to address elbow pain and injuries.

- Shoulder Point: The shoulder point is situated at the superior part of the ear, just above the apex of the triangular fossa. Although it's more related to the shoulder, stimulating this point can indirectly influence elbow discomfort and issues.

- Wrist Point: Located at the end of the helix's antihelix, the wrist point corresponds to the wrist area. Since the wrist and elbow are interconnected in terms of movement and functionality, this point could provide relief for elbow injuries as well.

- Musculoskeletal Area: This point is positioned on the antitragus, near the middle of the ear. It's a general point for musculoskeletal problems and can be included in auricular treatments for elbow injuries.

- Point Zero: Located at the centre of the ear, this point is considered a "reset" point that can have a harmonizing effect on the body's energy. It's often used at the beginning or end of auricular treatments.

Conclusion

The anatomy and functional complexity of the elbow make it susceptible to conditions like tennis elbow, golfer's elbow, and elbow strain. These injuries often result from repetitive motions, overuse, or sudden trauma, leading to pain, inflammation, and limited mobility. Using acupuncture, local blood circulation improves, helping with the reduction of inflammation, promoting the delivery of nutrients to the injured tissues and the release of endorphins and other neurotransmitters during acupuncture which contributes to pain relief and relaxation.

References

1. www.sciencedirect.com/topics/neuroscience/common-extensor-tendon.
2. Nirschl RP, Pettrone FA. Tennis elbow. The surgical treatment of lateral epicondylitis. J Bone Joint Surg Am. 1979.
3. McCarroll JR, Rettig AC, Shelbourne KD. Injuries in the Amateur Golfer.Phys Sportsmed.1990.
4. McHardy A, et al. American Journal of Sports Medicine, 2007, Aug. 35(8)

Chapter 13

Part 1 – Wrist Anatomy

The wrist joint which connects the hand to the forearm, is a complex assembly of bones, ligaments, tendons, and muscles which not only facilitates the flexible movement of the hand but also plays a fundamental role in enabling a wide range of daily activities, from delicate precision tasks to forceful actions. The wrist joint allows for movements, including flexion of 60 to 80 degrees, extension of 60 to 80 degrees, radial deviation of 20 degrees and ulnar deviation of 20 degrees.[1]

In sports, the wrist provides a junction where precision and power, come together. Whether it's the precise control required in a golf swing, the explosive force harnessed during a tennis serve, or the delicate manoeuvres of a gymnast, the wrist's function is essential in upper body sports. Given the abundance of bones, ligaments, tendons, and joints involved in the functioning of hands and wrists, there is a significant potential for injury. Injuries to the hand and wrists represent some of the most prevalent conditions affecting athletes. As about 25% of sports-related injuries pertain to the hand or wrist,[2] it is worth understanding sports related movements which occur at the wrist, as below.

Sports-Specific Movements at the Wrist

- In racquet sports such as tennis, badminton, squash, and table tennis, the wrist is vital in generating power and control during forehand and backhand swings.

- Gymnastic routines involve weight-bearing activities such as handstands and vaulting, rely on wrist strength, flexibility, and stability to support body weight and perform complex manoeuvres.

- Wrist strength and stability are crucial in rock climbing and bouldering. The flexor and extensor muscles around the wrist help maintain grip strength, stabilise the body, and control movements while climbing.

- In weightlifting, wrist stability and mobility are essential in movements like snatches, cleans, and overhead presses. They enable efficient weight support and force transfer from the body to the barbell.

- Wrist flexibility, stability, and strength are fundamental for striking, blocking, and grappling in martial arts and combat sports like boxing and judo.

The Structure of the Wrist Joint

The wrist joint, also called the radiocarpal joint, is a condyloid synovial joint of the distal upper limb that connects and serves as a transition point between the forearm and hand. A condyloid joint is a modified ball and socket joint that allows flexion, extension, abduction, and adduction movements.[3]

The radius, one of the two forearm bones, forms the primary articulation with the wrist's carpal bones. The ulna, the second forearm bone, does not directly contribute to wrist joint articulation but provides support to stabilise the wrist. There are eight carpal bones, organised into two rows, four in each row, progressing from the lateral (thumb) to the medial side (little finger);

- Proximal row: Scaphoid, Lunate, Triquetrum, Pisiform

- Distal row: Trapezium, Trapezoid, Capitate, Hamate

The end of the radius connects with the proximal row of carpal bones. At the same time, the ulna contributes through a fibrocartilaginous disc known as the triangular fibrocartilage complex, providing additional support to the wrist joint.

The joint is formed through the articulations between the distal radius and the scaphoid, lunate, and triquetrum. The proximal articulation forms a concave shape composed of a combination of the distal end of the radius and the articular disk. The distal articulation is convex and composed of the proximal hand's scaphoid, lunate, and triquetrum bones. Note that the ulna is not part of the wrist joint itself.

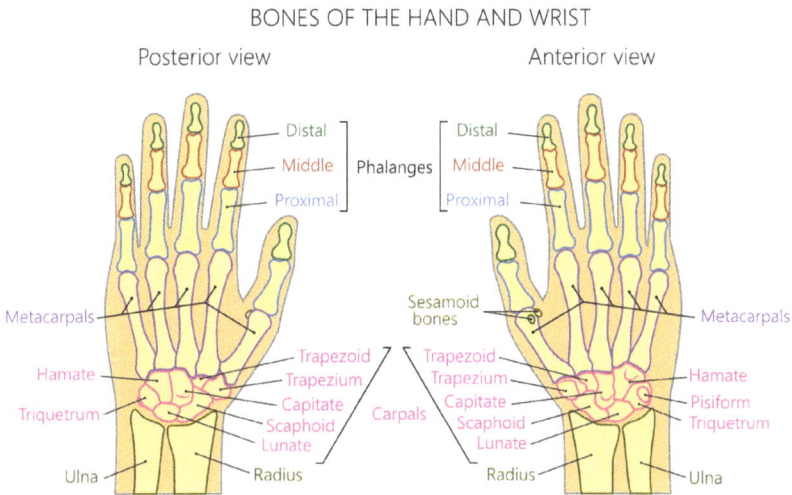

BONES OF THE HAND AND WRIST

Bones Wrist and hand Joint

Ligaments of the Wrist

The wrist joint is primarily supported and stabilised by four ligaments, each contributing to the joint's functionality and preventing unwanted movements. These ligaments play a critical role in enabling a wide range of hand and wrist motions while maintaining the structural integrity of the joint.

- **Palmar radiocarpal ligament:** Positioned on the anterior (palmar) aspect of the wrist joint, this ligament extends from the radius bone to both rows of carpal bones. Apart from enhancing the stability of the wrist, its primary function is to ensure that the hand moves in synchronisation with the forearm during supination, where the hand and forearm rotate outward.

- **Dorsal radiocarpal ligament:** Located on the wrist joint's posterior (dorsal) side, this ligament connects the radius bone to both rows of carpal bones. It plays a crucial role in maintaining the stability of the wrist joint.[4] Additionally, it facilitates coordinated movement between the hand and forearm during pronation, where the hand and forearm rotate inward.

- **Ulnar collateral ligament**: Runs from the ulnar styloid process to the triquetrum and pisiform bones. This ligament acts as a vital stabiliser of the wrist joint. Its primary function is to prevent excessive radial (lateral) deviation of the hand, helping to maintain proper alignment during various wrist movements.

- **Radial collateral ligament**: Extending from the radial styloid process to the scaphoid and trapezium bones, this ligament is essential for stabilising the wrist joint. Its primary role is to prevent excessive ulnar (medial) deviation of the hand, ensuring the wrist maintains proper alignment during different movements.

Wrist Muscles

Multiple muscles perform essential roles at the wrist joint in regulating movement and also providing stability. These muscles are primarily situated in the forearm but extend into the hand, enabling intricate motions of the wrist and fingers.

The main Flexors of the wrist are:

- **Flexor Carpi Radialis**: This muscle runs along the palmar side of the forearm, originating from the medial epicondyle of the humerus and attaching to the base of the second metacarpal bone. Its primary function involves flexing and abducting the hand at the wrist joint.

- **Flexor Carpi Ulnaris:** Located on the ulnar (inner) side of the forearm, this muscle originates from the medial epicondyle of the humerus and the olecranon process of the ulna. It inserts into the pisiform bone and the base of the fifth metacarpal. The flexor carpi ulnaris is responsible for flexing and adducting the hand at the wrist joint.

- **Palmaris Longus:** Positioned in the anterior forearm, this muscle runs from the medial epicondyle of the humerus to the palmar aponeurosis, a thick connective tissue in the palm. The presence of palmaris longus varies among individuals. Its role is to tense the palmar aponeurosis and aid in wrist flexion.

The main Extensors of the wrist are:

- **Extensor Carpi Radialis Longus and Brevis:** Found on the dorsal (back) side of the forearm, the extensor carpi radialis longus originates from the lateral supracondylar ridge of the humerus, while the extensor carpi radialis brevis originates from the lateral epicondyle of the humerus. Both muscles insert into the base of the second and third metacarpal bones. They are responsible for extending and abducting the hand at the wrist joint.

- **Extensor Carpi Ulnaris:** Situated on the posterior side of the forearm, this muscle arises from the lateral epicondyle of the humerus and the posterior border of the ulna. It inserts into the base of the fifth metacarpal bone. The extensor carpi ulnaris functions to extend and adduct the hand at the wrist joint.

- **Extensor Digitorum:** Situated on the posterior forearm, the extensor digitorum originates from the lateral epicondyle of the humerus and the posterior surface of the ulna. Extending into the fingers' dorsal expansion (extensor expansion), it allows for extension at the metacarpophalangeal and proximal interphalangeal joints and wrist extension.

Muscles of the Forearm
(right arm)

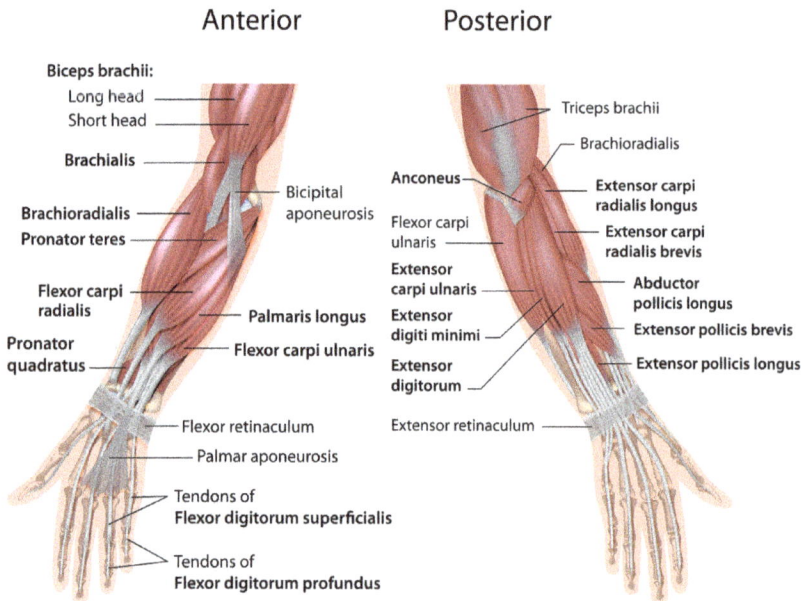

Anterior   Posterior

Biceps brachii:
Long head
Short head
Brachialis
Brachioradialis
Pronator teres
Bicipital aponeurosis
Flexor carpi radialis
Pronator quadratus
Palmaris longus
Flexor carpi ulnaris
Flexor retinaculum
Palmar aponeurosis
Tendons of Flexor digitorum superficialis
Tendons of Flexor digitorum profundus

Triceps brachii
Brachioradialis
Anconeus
Flexor carpi ulnaris
Extensor carpi ulnaris
Extensor digiti minimi
Extensor digitorum
Extensor retinaculum
Extensor carpi radialis longus
Extensor carpi radialis brevis
Abductor pollicis longus
Extensor pollicis brevis
Extensor pollicis longus

Right muscles of the forearm

There are two main groups of muscles that create finger movements, the extrinsic muscles and the intrinsic muscles. The extrinsic muscles originate outside the hand and have tendons that extend into the hand to control finger movements. They are responsible for gross movements of the fingers. The intrinsic muscles are located within the hand itself and are responsible for fine and precise movements of the fingers. They control individual finger motions.

Conclusion

The wrist anatomy enables a delicate equilibrium between stability and a wide range of motion. The arrangement of bones, ligaments, tendons, and soft tissues forms a synovial joint, facilitating diverse hand functions from fine motor skills to strong grips. Nevertheless, the wrist's flexibility which allows a wide range of motion, exposes it to injuries like sprains, strains, and conditions such as carpal tunnel syndrome.

References

1. https://www.livestrong.com/article/93432-normal-range-motion-wrist.
2. www:physiopedia.com. Hand and Wrist Sports Injuries.
3. Kauer JM. Functional anatomy of the wrist. Clin Orthop Relat Res. 1980 Jun.
4. Lewis OJ, Hamshere RJ, Bucknill TM. The anatomy of the wrist joint. J Anat. 1970 May;106

Chapter 13

Part 2 – Wrist Injuries and TCM Treatment

Wrist injuries in sports can manifest in various ways, often linked to the challenging physical demands and repetitive motions inherent to specific activities. Direct impact or trauma, prevalent in contact sports like football and martial arts, can result in fractures, sprains, or contusions. Overuse injuries of the wrist are common in sports involving repetitive wrist movements, such as tennis or weightlifting, potentially leading to conditions like tendinitis. Sudden, forceful actions like blocking a basketball shot or performing gymnastic routines can cause sprains or strains. Inadequate equipment or technique can increase the risk, while sports involving hyperextension or repetitive impacts, such as boxing, pose their own set of wrist injury challenges.

Commonly occurring wrist injuries are described below.

Wrist Tendinitis

Wrist tendinitis or tenosynovitis, is a condition characterised by inflammation and irritation of the wrist tendons. Wrist tendinitis caused by sports injuries, is the inflammation and irritation of the wrist tendons due to excessive use, repetitive movements, or traumatic incidents during sports activities. Tendinitis occurs when the synovial sheath surrounding the tendons becomes inflamed, leading to discomfort and pain in the affected area.

Sports that involve repetitive wrist movements, forceful gripping, or impact on the wrist joint increase the risk of developing tendinitis. Activities like tennis, golf, weightlifting, gymnastics, and racquet sports are particularly prone to causing wrist tendinitis. Athletes in these sports often subject their wrists to repeated motions or strain, resulting in wear and tear on the tendons and synovial sheaths.

Wrist tendonitis can be considered in TCM as a *Jin Gu Syndrome*, characterised by pain, stiffness and limited range of motion in the tendons, ligaments and joints, accompanied by swelling and inflammation.

Symptoms of wrist tenosynovitis in sports injuries include:

- Pain in the wrist joint, ranging from a dull ache to sharp pain, and may worsen with specific wrist movements or activities.

- The inflammation of tendons and synovial sheaths can cause swelling around the wrist area.

- The wrist may feel stiff, making it challenging for athletes to move their wrists freely.

- The affected wrist becomes tender to the touch, especially over the inflamed tendons.

- Wrist tendinitis can weaken the hand, impacting grip strength and overall hand function.

An example of wrist tendinitis is **De Quervain's tenosynovitis** which primarily affects two tendons; the abductor pollicis longus and the extensor pollicis brevis. These tendons are responsible for palm abduction and extension.

The exact cause of De Quervain's tenosynovitis is not always apparent, but it is often associated with repetitive thumb movements or activities that strain the tendons.[1] Engaging in repetitive lifting, gripping, and twisting motions can lead to irritation and inflammation of the tendons and the protective sheath surrounding them. The condition is not so common in sports but is more prevalent in certain occupations and hobbies that involve repetitive thumb motions, such as gardening, carpentry, and playing musical instruments.

DE QUERVAIN'S TENOSYNOVITIS

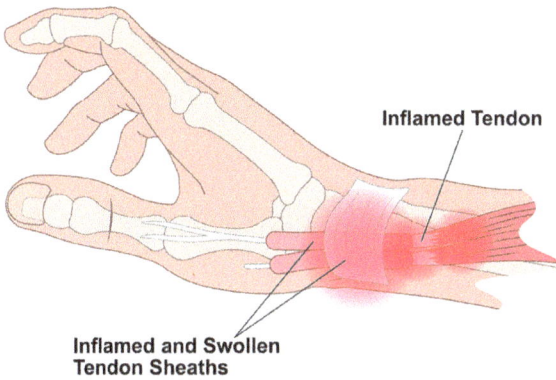

Inflamed Tendon

Inflamed and Swollen Tendon Sheaths

De Quervain's

Carpal Tunnel Syndrome

The carpal tunnel is a narrow, rigid passageway formed by the wrist bones and a tough band of tissue called the transverse carpal ligament.[2] The repetitive motions or overuse of the wrist and hand can lead to irritation and inflammation of the tendons in the wrist, which can compress the median nerve, which passes through the carpal tunnel.

Carpal tunnel syndrome is normally associated with sports and musculoskeletal injuries, particularly those involving repetitive motions or prolonged use of the hands and wrists in sports such as tennis, golf, weightlifting, and racquetball. However, only some people participating in these activities will develop carpal tunnel syndrome, and other factors such as ergonomics, posture, and individual susceptibility may also play a role.

Apart from repetitive motion and prolonged use of hands and wrist, there are risk factors which may contribute to the syndrome. One such example is that some individuals may have a naturally smaller carpal tunnel or other anatomical variations that make them more prone to developing carpal tunnel syndrome. Also, hormonal changes during pregnancy can lead to fluid retention and swelling, increasing pressure within the carpal tunnel and compressing the median nerve.[3] Certain medical conditions, such as rheumatoid arthritis,

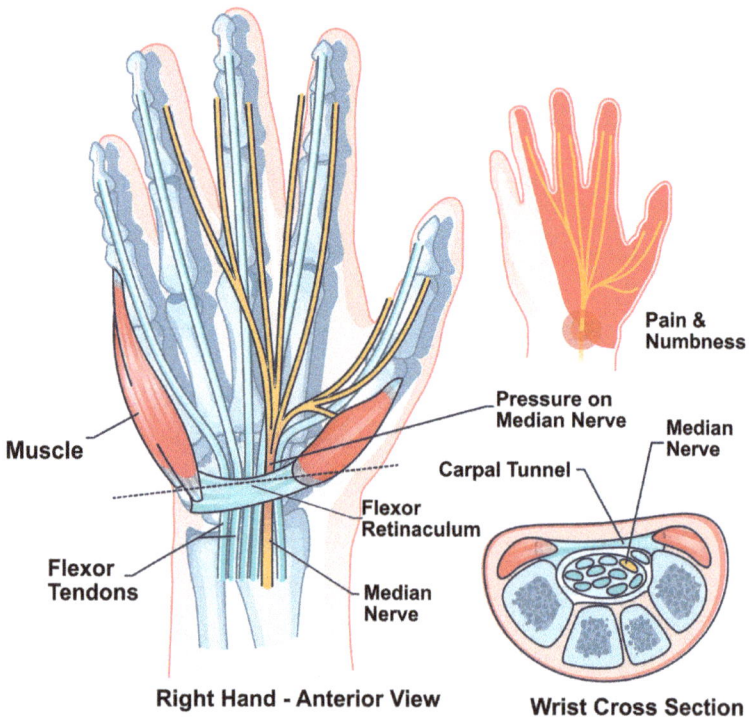

Carpal Tunnel Syndrome

diabetes, thyroid dysfunction, and hormonal imbalances, can increase the risk of developing carpal tunnel syndrome.

Symptoms of Carpal Tunnel Syndrome (CTS):

- A characteristic indication of carpal tunnel syndrome is a sensation of numbness and tingling, often likened to pins and needles, in the thumb, index finger, middle finger, and part of the ring finger. This feeling can extend into the hand and even up to the forearm.

- CTS can result in hand weakness, making tasks like gripping objects, delicate motor activities, or maintaining a firm hold more challenging. Some patients might describe a sensation of burning in the hand and fingers affected by CTS.

- Pain and discomfort in the hand and wrist, which can radiate from the wrist to the arm. This pain might fluctuate or remain constant, intensifying during actions that involve wrist and hand use.

- Discomfort or pain might be present around the wrist area, sometimes extending to the forearm.

- Swelling or mild puffiness around the wrist can manifest, especially in cases of chronic or severe CTS.

- In certain instances, the affected hand or fingers might feel abnormally cold due to compromised nerve function.

- Tasks necessitating precision, such as fastening buttons or typing, can become more arduous due to weakened grip and diminished sensation caused by CTS.

- Activities involving repetitive wrist movements or extended wrist bending, like keyboard typing or using a computer mouse, can worsen CTS symptoms.

Acupuncture can be particularly useful in treating Carpal Tunnel Syndrome. Acupuncture points for carpal tunnel syndrome depend on the individual's symptoms and underlying imbalances but points below may be beneficial;

- **PC6:** Located inside the forearm, about two finger-widths above the wrist crease, between the tendons. It alleviates pain, reduces inflammation, and promotes relaxation.

- **PC7:** Found on the palmar surface of the wrist, approximately in line with the middle finger. This point is often used to treat CTS-related pain and numbness.

- **SJ4:** Located on the back of the hand, in the depression between the knuckles of the ring finger and little finger when bent. Relieves wrist and hand pain.

- **SJ5:** Situated on the back of the forearm, about two finger-widths above the wrist crease, between the tendons. They are frequently used to treat CTS, specifically to alleviate pain and improve hand function.

- **LI4:** Located on the back of the hand, in the webbing between the thumb and index finger. LI4 is a versatile acupuncture point commonly used for pain relief and promoting energy flow.

- **PC3:** Located on the palmar surface of the forearm, in the depression between the tendons of the palmaris longus and flexor carpi radialis muscles, often used to relieve pain and numbness associated with CTS.

- **LI10:** Found on the radial side of the forearm, between the tendons of the extensor carpi radialis longus and brevis muscles, reducing wrist and hand pain.

- **TE3:** Located on the dorsum of the hand, in the depression between the fourth and fifth metacarpal bones. Relieves pain and promotes circulation in the hand.

- **TE10:** Found on the dorsum of the forearm, about two finger-widths above the wrist crease, between the ulna and radius bones. Used for wrist and forearm pain associated with CTS.

Wrist Strain and Sprain

Wrist sprains and wrist strains are often used interchangeably, as they have similar symptoms. Both involve damage to the soft tissues around the wrist joint, such as muscles, tendons, and ligaments, but they differ in the specific tissues affected and the mechanism of injury. Distinguishing between an injury as a sprain or a strain offers understanding into the expected recovery timeline and the potential for long-term issues. Ligaments typically heal more slowly than muscles or tendons. Also, addressing or treating a sprain often involves focusing more on stabilizing the wrist joint, while managing a strain could require exercises aimed at strengthening the affected muscles or tendons.

Wrist Sprains

Wrist sprains occur when the ligaments in the wrist are subjected to excessive force or stretching beyond their normal range of motion and involve various ligaments around the wrist joint and also ligaments which connect the bones of the hand. The ligaments affected are;

- Scapholunate Ligament which connects the scaphoid and lunate bones. Sprains to this ligament are quite common and can result from falls on an outstretched hand.

- Radiocarpal Ligaments connect the radius bone to various carpal bones. They help stabilize the wrist joint and can be sprained due to impacts or excessive movement.

- Ulnar Collateral Ligament which stabilizes the ulnar side of the wrist can be sprained during excessive ulnar deviation.

- Radial Collateral Ligament stabilizes the radial side of the wrist and can be sprained during excessive radial deviation

- Palmar Radiocarpal Ligaments run on the palmar side of the wrist and contribute to its stability. They can be sprained during hyperextension or hyperflexion of the wrist.

- Dorsal Radiocarpal Ligaments, on the dorsal side of the wrist, plays a role in preventing excessive wrist flexion. They can be sprained due to hyperextension or sudden impacts.

- Interosseous Ligaments which connect the carpal bones to each other can also be affected by sprains.

- Triangular Fibrocartilage Complex (TFCC), is composed of ligaments, cartilage, and other soft tissues, stabilizes the ulnar side of the wrist. TFCC sprains can occur due to sudden twisting motions or repetitive loading.

Similar to other sprains, symptoms of a sprained wrist include pain which may be felt at the site of the injury and radiate throughout the wrist area. Other symptoms include, swelling, bruising, stiffness and weakness of the wrist.

Wrist Strain

A wrist strain is an injury that involves the stretching or tearing of muscles or tendons in the wrist area. As with wrist sprains, wrist strains typically occur due to sudden or excessive force applied to the wrist, often resulting from activities that involve repetitive motions or overuse.

Examples of sports where wrist strains may occur:

- Tennis players often experience wrist strains, especially during powerful serves or when hitting backhands. The repetitive swinging motion can strain the wrist tendons.

- Golfers can develop wrist strains, particularly if they have an improper swing technique or grip. The impact of hitting the ball can also stress the wrist.

- Weightlifters may experience wrist strains when lifting heavy weights, especially during exercises like bench presses, overhead presses, or clean and jerk movements.

- Gymnasts put a lot of stress on their wrists, especially when performing handstands, flips, or other intricate manoeuvres on the uneven bars, rings, or floor exercises.

Wrist strains typically affect muscles and tendons, around the wrist joint. The primary muscles involved in wrist strains include:

- Flexor muscles, including the flexor carpi radialis, flexor carpi ulnaris, and palmaris longus

- Extensor muscles which are the extensor carpi radialis brevis, extensor carpi radialis longus, and extensor carpi ulnaris.

- Pronator muscles, these muscles are responsible for pronating or turning the palm downward. The pronator teres and pronator quadratus are two muscles that play a role in wrist movement.

- Supinator muscle, along with the biceps brachii, assists in supination of the forearm and wrist.

Symptoms of a wrist sprain and a wrist strain are quite similar because they both involve injury to the soft tissues around the wrist. Common symptoms that both conditions share are:

- Both wrist sprains and strains typically cause pain in the affected area. The pain can range from mild to severe, depending on the extent of the injury.

- Swelling is a common response to tissue damage, and it can occur with both sprains and strains. The affected area may appear puffy or swollen.

- Blood vessels may rupture as a result of the injury, leading to bruising around the wrist.

- Both conditions can restrict the normal range of motion of the wrist.

- The area around the wrist may feel tender to the touch due to inflammation and tissue damage.

- There is a sense of weakness in the wrist, making it challenging to perform tasks that involve gripping or lifting.

- Both conditions can lead to stiffness in the wrist joint, making it uncomfortable to move.

- With wrist strain there might be muscle spasms or cramps in the forearm or hand.

Triangular Fibrocartilage Complex

- The Triangular Fibrocartilage Complex (TFCC) is a structure located in the wrist and participates in movements that involve rotation or gripping. TFCC consist of cartilage, ligaments, tendons, and other soft tissues that are situated on the ulnar side of the wrist. The components of TFCC include articular discs, the ulnar collateral and the radioulnar ligaments. Tendons of various muscles that control wrist and finger movements pass through or attach to the TFCC.

- TFCC's function is to stabilize the wrist joint and prevent excessive rotational movement and provides a cushioning effect, distributing forces and reducing friction within the wrist joint.

- TFCC injuries can result from various causes, including trauma, overuse, and degeneration. Most of the symptoms, such as pain, swelling and wrist stiffness can lead to a feeling of wrist instability on the ulnar side, making the wrist feel weak or unreliable during activities.

- Factors such as wrist injuries, trauma or impact, repetitive stress and normal wear and tear can contribute to wrist instability.

TFCC
TRIANGULAR FIBROCARTILAGE COMPLEX

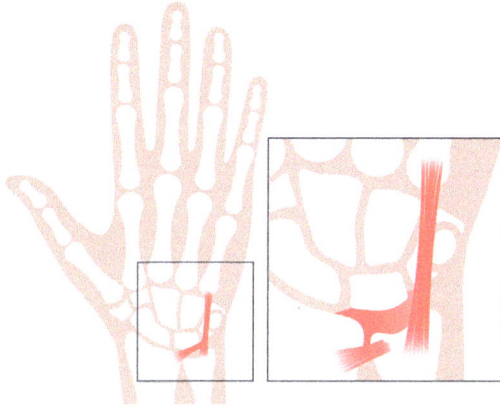

TFCC

TCM Treatment of the Wrist

In Traditional Chinese Medicine, wrist sports injuries can be traced back to various underlying causes and factors. These injuries occur due to imbalances in the flow of Qi and Blood, influenced by both external and internal elements. Physical trauma and overexertion during sports activities disrupt the natural flow of Qi and Blood, leading to stagnation and injury. The force of trauma from an injury can take many forms, such as wrenching, impact, compression, and stretching of the muscle, tendon, or ligaments, causing classical signs of inflammation, pain, redness, swelling, and heat. Other causes of wrist sports injuries include external pathogens like Wind, Cold, Heat, or Dampness, which can weaken the wrist's protective Wei Qi, making it more susceptible to injury. Treatment of wrist injuries, with acupuncture is therefore based on addressing the above.

During the acute stage of trauma, that is the first seventy-two hours, acupuncture treatment using local points is not advised as needling could exacerbate the inflammatory response and also be painful for the patient. During this stage, "PRICE" (Protect, Rest, Ice, Compression and Elevation) is advised. For pain relief, wrist/ankle points, as below could be used as well as other distal points, choosing points which help with inflammation and pain relief. Auricular points such as Shenmen, Thalamus, Adrenal, Endocrine as well as the wrist point would be beneficial.

Wrist/Ankle points

- HT7 to KID3, PC7 to LR4, LU9 to SP5, LI5 to ST41, SJ4 to GB40, SI4 to BL62

Local and Adjacent Points for wrist injuries

Please see Appendix 1 for Acupuncture Point Location.

- **SJ4:** Relaxes sinews and alleviates pain. Beneficial for subacute conditions when the wrist is weak and there is redness, swelling and pain. It can be combined with LI11 and LI4 if there is stiffness in the fingers.

  Needling: 0.3cun to 0.5cun, slightly oblique insertion towards the radius.

- **SJ5:** Activates the channel and also alleviates pain. Useful point for expelling, especially wind-damp Bi. Clears heat. Combine with LI5 and LI11 if fingers and elbows are affected. Can be used instead of SJ4

  Needling: 0.5cun to 1.0cun. Oblique insertion towards the ulna. Caution: After insertion, patient movement can result in needle bending

- **LI5:** Benefits wrist joint. Clears Heat and alleviates pain. A useful point when the elbow is also affected.

  Needling: 0.5cun to 1cun, perpendicular—caution: cephalic vein.

- **SI4:** Activates channel and alleviates pain. Clears heat and reduces swelling, a useful point in the early stages of subacute injury. Used when fingers, elbows and neck are affected (along the channel).

  Needling: 0.3cun – 0.5cun, perpendicular.

- **SI5:** Clears Heat and reduces swelling (used as an adjacent point). Useful in early subacute and also when the shoulder is affected, combined with BL36, BL40 and BL56, and if the elbow is affected, use LI11

  Needling: 0.3cun – 0.5cun, perpendicular

- **PC7:** Used when thumb and wrist are affected (De Quervain's Syndrome) and for carpal tunnel syndrome.

  Needling: 0.3cun – 0.5cun perpendicular. Caution: Median nerve.

- **LU7:** Pacifies wind and releases exterior Bi. Strengthens Wei Qi and frees connecting channel (to open pores). Activates the Lung channel and alleviates pain. Useful point when there is pain of the thumb

  Needling: 0.3cun – 0.5cun; pinch the skin and insert the needle obliquely upwards.

Additional points which can be used:

- Outer and Inner gate: P6 + SJ 5 and four gates: Liv3 +LI 4, bilaterally.
- SI5 and H7 when there is a limitation of movement
- SI4 and SJ5 if numbness is present.

Distal Points

Normally Distal points are chosen because of their clinical significance and also because of their relationship to the points being used locally. *However, the wrist does not have any true distal points.* The upper and lower corresponding points for the Wrist/Ankle mentioned above can be used to overcome this. The meridian affected should be identified when treating wrist injuries, as this determines the acupuncture points to use. For example, if the pain is along the anterior aspect of the wrist, then points along the Lung channel are chosen. If pain is along the posterior aspect, then points along the Large Intestine Channel are chosen. In addition to wrist/ankle points, systemic distal body points can be used to alleviate pain and reduce inflammation.

The meridians around the wrist are:

- On the posterior aspect: San Jiao, Small Intestine and Large Intestinc (yang channel)

- On the anterior aspect: Lung, Heart and Pericardium (yin channel)

For wrist injuries, depending on the meridian affected, following distal points can be used:

- If the Small Intestine channel is affected, use **BL60.**

- If the Large Intestine channel is affected, **ST41.**

- If the San Jiao channel is affected, use **GB40.**

- If the Lung channel is affected, use **SP5.**

- If the Pericardium channel is affected, use **Liv4.**

- If the Heart channel affected **Kid3.**

Other Points to Alleviate Pain and Reduce Inflammation:

SP10: Located on the inner thigh, about three finger-widths above the knee. SP10 can be used to clear Heat and Dampness, making it useful for resolving inflammation.

LI4: Located on the back of the hand, in the webbing between the thumb and index finger. LI4 is a useful point used for pain relief and reducing inflammation throughout the body.

ST36: Located on the lower leg, about four finger-widths below the kneecap and one finger-width towards the outside of the leg, ST36 can strengthen the body's overall Qi and can be beneficial for recovery from injuries.

GB34: Located on the outer side of the lower leg, just below the knee, can help reduce inflammation and alleviate pain.

SP6: Located on the inner side of the lower leg, about four finger-widths above the ankle. SP6 can be used to promote blood circulation and reduce swelling.

Wrist Pain due to Painful Obstruction Syndrome (Bi)

- When the wrist has *Wandering Bi*, the pathogen is Wind. Typically, the pain may migrate in the wrist from one location to another, such as the elbow or from anterior to posterior. The pain may be felt more in windy conditions. The athlete may also suffer from chills and have a mild fever.

  Tongue: Normal body with a thin white coat.

  Pulse: Wiry.

  Acupuncture points: BL12, BL17, SP10 or DU16; points which promote Blood and so eliminate Wind.

- If the wrist suffers from *fixed, stabbing-like pain*, which is often quite severe, this is likely to be caused by the dominating Cold pathogenic factor, compared to Wind or Damp pathogen. The pain of Cold Bi is often alleviated by warmth but aggravated by cold. Soft tissues around the wrist may also feel tight, and the joint feel stiff.

For cold Bi, mostly deep needling is used with moxa.

Tongue: Normal body with a thin white coat.

Pulse: Tight.

Acupuncture points: BL23, CV4 or Ren4. Warms Kidney strengthens Yang, and so eliminates Cold.

- If the wrist feels *heavy and sore*, the chief pathogenic factor is Damp and is called Fixed Bi. The area around the wrist may also feel numb. There may also be swelling of the wrist, which should not be confused with swelling that follows acute injury due to the inflammatory response. Fixed Bi is marked by heaviness and numbness. Fixed Bi is often aggravated by damp and rainy weather. Moxa is also helpful.

Tongue: Normal body with white and greasy coating.

Pulse: Soft, slow and can be slippery.

Acupuncture points: SP 6, SP 9, GB 34 or ST 36 strengthens Spleen and eliminates Dampness.

- Heat Bi typically causes *redness and swelling* in the affected joints and is associated with inflammation. The joint pain in Heat Bi is often sharp, intense, and burning in nature. It may be aggravated by heat or pressure and may be relieved by cold applications. The joints may appear warm to the touch.

Tongue is red or deep red, with a thin or absent coating.

Pulse is rapid, feel full and forceful.

Acupuncture points for clearing Heat Bi include, LI11, LI4 (especially useful for hands, wrist and fingers), LI2, ST36, SI3 and LI5.

Conclusion

Wrist injuries often results in pain, stiffness, and limited mobility. By carefully selecting acupuncture points along relevant meridians, TCM practitioner can influence the flow of Qi, Blood and elimination of pathogenic factors from the injured wrist, promoting the body's natural healing processes. Local points near the wrist, adjacent points along the meridian pathways, and distal points away from the injury site are strategically chosen based on TCM diagnosis and pattern differentiation. These acupuncture points serve to alleviate pain, reduce inflammation, and restore balance to the wrist joint. They also play a crucial role in addressing the underlying TCM patterns that contribute to the injury, such as Qi stagnation, Blood stasis, Dampness, or Cold.

References

1. www.berkshirehealthcare.nhs.uk
2. Ozturk, Kahraman, et al. "Comparison of Carpal Tunnel Injection Techniques: A Cadaver Study." Scandinavian Journal of Plastic and Reconstructive Surgery and Hand Surgery, 2008
3. Humbyrd CJ, LaPorte DM. Hand surgery: considerations in pregnant patients. *J Hand Surg Am.* 2012

Chapter 14

Part 1 - Hip Anatomy

The hip joint is also called the acetabulofemoral joint. It is an important joint supporting the upper body and transferring weight of the upper body downwards to the ground, enabling actions like standing, walking, and running. It is also one of the most mobile joints in the human body, providing movement in all three planes of motion; sagittal, frontal, and transverse. The flexibility of the hip joint to carry out movements in all three planes is due to the structure of the joint, ligaments and the muscles supporting the hip joint. The intricate structure also provides stability to the hip.

Hip Joint

The hip joint is the articulation of the femoral head and the acetabulum.

The femoral head is the rounded, ball-like end of the femur that articulates with the acetabulum. It is covered with articular cartilage, which helps reduce friction and distributes loads during movement. The femoral head is connected to the shaft of the femur by the femoral neck. It is oriented obliquely, contributing to the hip joint's range of motion. The angle of inclination and anteversion of the femoral neck can vary among individuals, affecting the overall mechanics of the hip joint.

The acetabulum is a deep, cup-shaped socket on the lateral surface of the pelvis, formed by the fusion of three bones; the ilium, ischium, and pubis. It is lined with articular cartilage, thicker at the superior and anterior regions, providing more stability to the joint in weight-bearing positions. The acetabular labrum is a fibrocartilaginous ring that lines the rim of the acetabulum. It deepens the socket, providing more stability to the hip joint and enhancing the femoral head's fit within the acetabulum. The labrum is crucial in distributing forces evenly across the hip joint surface during activities like walking, running, or standing, reducing pressure on specific points and protecting the cartilage. Moreover, the labrum assists shock absorption during weight-bearing movements, effectively reducing the impact forces transmitted through the hip joint. This is especially important for athletes and individuals engaging in high-impact activities. The labrum also contributes to joint lubrication by efficiently distributing synovial fluid within the hip joint. Labral tears can result from various factors, including trauma, repetitive stress, or anatomical abnormalities, and may necessitate medical attention or surgical intervention to restore proper joint function.

Synovial membrane, which forms the inner lining of the joint capsule, produces synovial fluid, a viscous liquid that lubricates the joint surfaces, reducing friction during movement. The synovial fluid also supplies nutrients to the articular cartilage, aiding in nourishment and maintenance.

The hip joint is enclosed by a strong fibrous capsule that surrounds the joint and attaches to the edges of the acetabulum and the femoral neck.[1] This capsule helps stabilize the joint and contains synovial fluid.

Hip Ligaments

Ligaments play a vital role at the hip joint ensuring stability and controlling excessive movements. The main ligaments found in the hip joint are:

- **The Iliofemoral Ligament**: The body's strongest ligament in terms of its tensile strength. It is also called the Ligament of Bigelow. The primary function is to prevent excessive extension of the hip joint. Acting as a critical stabilizer, especially when standing upright, the ligament helps maintain an erect posture by resisting hyperextension of the hip. Originates from the pelvis at two points: the anterior inferior iliac spine and the superior acetabular rim. It attaches to the femur's intertrochanteric line, a ridge on the front surface of the femur.

- **The Pubofemoral Ligament:** Its primary function is to limit excessive abduction (outward movement) and extension of the hip joint. It contributes to hip stability during activities involving leg swinging or pivoting motions. Originates from the superior pubic ramus, the upper part of the pubic bone. It attaches to the proximal part of the femur, just below the lesser trochanter, and blends with the hip joint capsule.

- **Ischiofemoral Ligament**: Restricts excessive internal rotation of the hip joint. It plays a crucial role in maintaining joint stability and preventing over-rotation of the femoral head within the acetabulum. The ligament originates from the ischium, particularly from the ischial part of the acetabular rim. It attaches to the posterior part of the femur's neck, close to the greater trochanter, and merges with the joint capsule.

- **Ligamentum Teres**: Also known as the Round Ligament, has a relatively minor role in hip joint stability compared to other ligaments. It does, however, help in stabilizing the hip joint, particularly during rotational and lateral movements. The Ligamentum Teres originates from the acetabular notch and attaches to the fovea capitis, a slight depression on the femoral head.

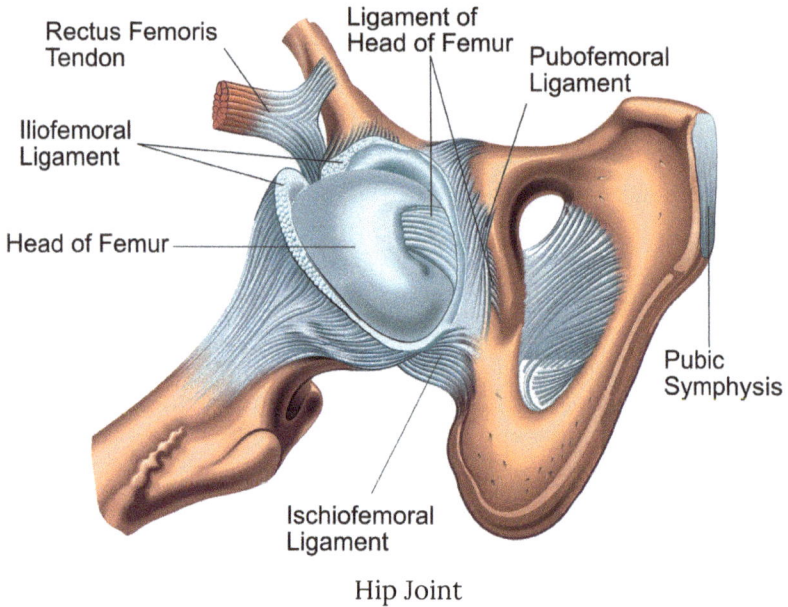

RIGHT HIP JOINT AND ASSOCIATED LIGAMENTS

Rectus Femoris Tendon

Ligament of Head of Femur

Pubofemoral Ligament

Iliofemoral Ligament

Head of Femur

Pubic Symphysis

Ischiofemoral Ligament

Hip Joint

Hip Muscles

The hip and upper leg region is a complex anatomical area containing many muscles contributing to various movements and functions. While the exact number of muscles can vary depending on how individual muscles are classified and whether more minor or less prominent muscles are included, there are over fifteen major muscles in this region. For this book's purpose, the muscles below are described in terms of their function.

Hip Flexors

The hip flexors are a group of muscles located in the front of the hip and upper thigh that work together to flex the hip joint. The main muscles that form the hip flexors include:

Iliopsoas: This is a combination of two muscles, the psoas major and the iliacus, that work together to flex the hip.

The iliacus originates from the iliac fossa of the ilium, while the psoas major originates from the vertebral body. Both muscles insert on the lesser trochanter of the femur.[2]

- **Rectus Femoris:** This is one of the four muscles that make up the quadriceps muscle group. It is the only one of the four that crosses both the hip and knee joints. It originates from the hip bone, that is the anterior inferior iliac spine and inserts on the patella and then continues to the tibia via the patellar tendon. Due to its attachment across the hip and the knee, it also extends the knee.[3]

- **Sartorius:** While the sartorius is primarily known for its role in flexing the knee, it also contributes to hip flexion. It runs obliquely across the front of the thigh, originating from the anterior superior iliac spine and inserting on the medial surface of the tibia near the knee. Sartorius is also the longest muscle found in the human body.

These muscles are crucial for various movements like walking, running, kicking, and lifting the leg. They play an important role in activities that involve lifting the thigh toward the chest or bringing the chest toward the thigh.

Hip Extensors

The primary muscles responsible for hip extension are:

- **Gluteus Maximus:** This is the largest and most powerful muscle in the buttocks. It originates from the posterior ilium, sacrum, and coccyx, and it inserts on the femur. The gluteus maximus is responsible for straightening and extending the hip joint.

- **Hamstrings:** While the primary function of the hamstrings is to flex the knee, they also play a role in extending the hip. The hamstrings are a group of three muscles located on the back of the thigh:

- Biceps Femoris has two heads, a long head and a short head. The long head originates from the ischial tuberosity (part of the pelvis) and the short head from linea aspera of the femur insert on the lateral aspect of the head of the fibula.

- Semimembranosus originates from the ischial tuberosity and inserts on the proximal medial condyle of the tibia.

- Semitendinosus, like the semimembranosus, this muscle also originates from the ischial tuberosity and inserts on the proximal end of tibia below medial condyle.

- Adductor Magnus: While the primary role of the adductor magnus is to adduct the thigh (bring it toward the midline of the body), it also plays a secondary role in hip extension. It originates from the ischial tuberosity and the lower part of the pubis and inserts on the linea aspera of the femur.

Hip Abductors

- The primary hip abductor is the Gluteus Medius which is located on the lateral side of the thigh, originating from the ilium and attaches to the greater trochanter of the femur. The gluteus medius also assists in stabilizing the pelvis during the stance phase of walking. The stance phase is the second phase of the gait cycle, during which the foot is in contact with the ground supporting the body's weight. The first phase is the swing phase, during which one leg moves through the air and does not make contact with the ground.

  Gluteus Minimus, Tensor Fasciae Latae and the Sartorius muscles also contribute to hip abduction.

Hip Adductors

- The hip adductors are the Adductor Brevis muscle and the Pectineus muscle. The adductor brevis muscle originates from the inferior pubic ramus and inserts into the femur's linea aspera, while the pectineus muscle originates from the superior pubic ramus and attaches to the pectineal line of the femur.

  The other muscles contributing to hip adduction are Adductor Longus, Adductor Magnus and the Gracilis muscle.

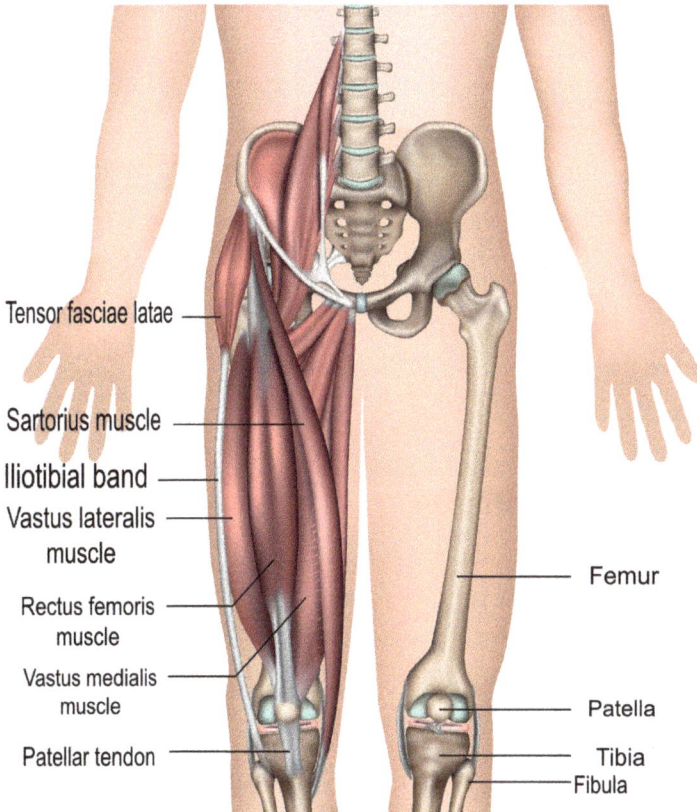

Anterior Thigh

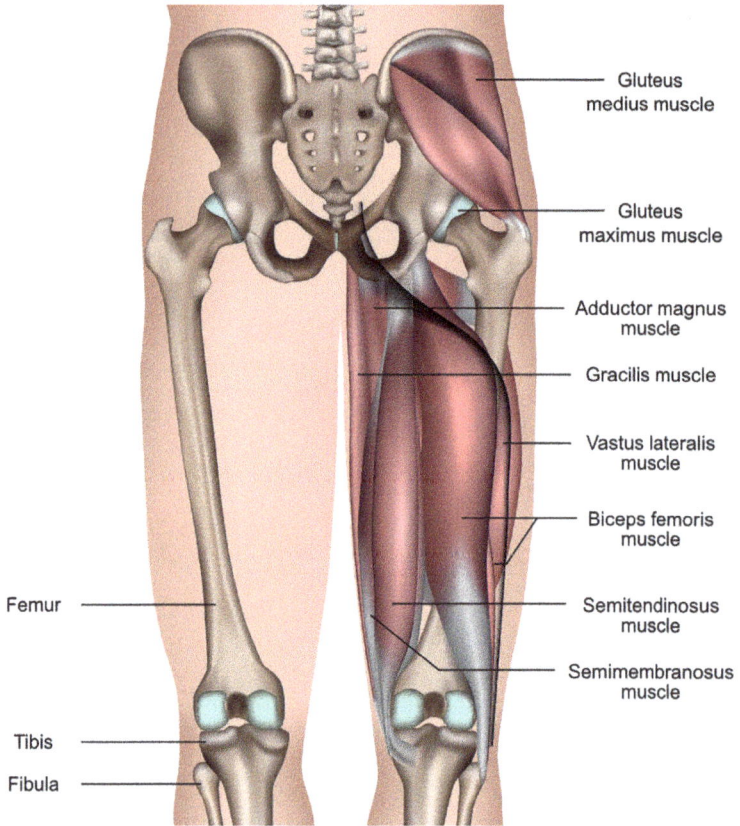

	Gluteus medius muscle
	Gluteus maximus muscle
	Adductor magnus muscle
	Gracilis muscle
	Vastus lateralis muscle
	Biceps femoris muscle
Femur	Semitendinosus muscle
	Semimembranosus muscle
Tibis	
Fibula	

Posterior Thigh

Hip External Rotators

External hip rotation is the movement of rotating the thigh outward from its normal anatomical position so that the front of the thigh moves away from the midline of the body and the toes point outward. This movement is important for maintaining balance, proper alignment, and adaptability while running.

- The hip external rotator is the Piriformis muscle which is deep in the gluteal region. It is a flat, pyramid-shaped muscle that originates from the sacrum's anterior surface and attaches to the upper border of the greater trochanter of the femur.

The other muscles which assist with external hip rotation are Gemellus Superior, Gemellus Inferior, Quadratus Femoris and Obturator Internus.

Hip Internal Rotators

Internal hip rotation is the action of rotating the thigh inwards, bringing the front of the thigh closer to the body's midline, a movement which occurs when crossing legs while seated.

- Muscles which internally rotate the hip include the Gluteus Medius, Gluteus Minimus, anterior fibres of the Gluteus Maximus and the Tensor Fasciae Latae.

Conclusion

The hip comprises of essential anatomical components that collectively contribute to its movement and functionality. Adding stability is the labrum, a cartilage structure. Central to this is the hip joint. Surrounding the joint are various muscles, including the robust hip flexors such as the iliopsoas, for hip flexion, and the gluteal muscles, enabling extension and sideways movement. Ligaments like the iliofemoral, pubofemoral, and ischiofemoral provide added stability and control. Together, these structures allow a broad array of motions, supporting activities from walking and jogging to leaping and turning, all while promoting overall stability and posture.

References

1. Hip joint: Bones, movements, muscles. Kenhub.
2. Iliopsoas: Origin, Insertion, Action & Nerve Supply. www: howtorelief.com/iliopsoas-origin-insertion-action-nerve-supply/
3. MuscleWiki - Simplify Your Workout. www:musclewiki.com/ muscle/quads.

Chapter 14

Part 2 – Hip Injuries and TCM Treatment

In sports, the hip plays a fundamental role by delivering stability, mobility, and strength to a variety of movements. It ensures balance and steadiness during weight-bearing tasks providing an extensive range of motion for dynamic actions. These actions include generating power for activities like jumping and sprinting, facilitating rapid directional changes, transferring forces between upper and lower body, and helps in absorbing impact. Hip muscles like the glutes, quadriceps, and hamstrings are pivotal for generating power in running, jumping, and striking movements. The hip's contribution in running entails coordinated extension and flexion, while in jumping, it assists in absorbing impact and creating force.

Hip and Upper Leg Sprains

A hip sprain occurs when the ligaments around the hip joint are stretched, torn, or damaged due to excessive force or movement. The severity of a hip sprain can vary, ranging from mild stretching of the ligaments to partial or complete tears. Common symptoms of a hip sprain include pain, swelling, limited range of motion, and difficulty bearing weight on the affected leg. In severe cases, the sprain can lead to significant instability in the hip joint.

Ligaments Affected in Hip Sprain (see previous diagram):

- **Iliofemoral Ligament:** The iliofemoral ligament is one of the strongest ligaments in the human body and plays a significant role in hip stability. It is situated on the front of the hip joint and prevents excessive extension of the hip, which could otherwise lead to overextension of the joint during activities like standing, walking, or running.

- **Pubofemoral Ligament:** Also found on the front side of the hip joint, the pubofemoral ligament connects the pubic bone to the femur. It helps prevent excessive abduction (movement away from the midline of the body) of the hip joint. This ligament provides stability during movements like leg swings and squatting.

- **Ischiofemoral Ligament:** Situated on the back side of the hip joint, the ischiofemoral ligament connects the ischium to the femur. It contributes to limiting excessive internal rotation of the hip joint, which is important for maintaining proper hip alignment during activities involving rotation of the leg.

Hip sprains are classified according to damage to the ligaments. There are three commonly used grades to classify sprains:

- **Grade 1 (Mild):** In a grade 1 sprain, the ligament is stretched but not torn. There might be some microscopic tearing of the ligament fibres, resulting in mild pain, swelling, and minimal joint instability. The joint's overall function is not severely affected.

- **Grade 2 (Moderate):** A grade 2 sprain involves a partial tear of the ligament fibres, resulting in more significant pain, swelling, and moderate joint instability. The affected joint might experience some loss of function, and there can be bruising.

- **Grade 3 (Severe):** A grade 3 sprain is the most severe and occurs when there is a complete ligament tear. This type of sprain leads to intense pain, significant swelling, and substantial joint instability with severe bruising.

Athletes participating in sports such as soccer, basketball, football, gymnastics, and martial arts are at a higher risk of experiencing hip sprains due to the nature of these activities. Additionally, runners and dancers might also be susceptible to hip sprains due to the repetitive and sometimes strenuous movements they perform.

Hip Sprain Symptoms:

- The pain from a hip sprain can range from a mild ache to severe discomfort, depending on the extent of ligament damage. The pain is often felt in the groin area or on the outside of the hip. Activities that involve hip movements, such as walking, running, squatting, or climbing stairs, can exacerbate the pain and discomfort.

- The hip joint might feel stiff and less flexible due to both the injury and the body's attempt to immobilize the area to protect it.

- Swelling around the hip joint may be felt after a sprain due to the body's inflammatory response. The affected area may feel warm to the touch in addition to appearing swollen or puffy.

- If the hip sprain was the result of direct impact or trauma, bruising might develop over time due to blood vessels breaking beneath the skin.

- Swelling, pain, and muscle spasm can lead to a reduced ability to move the hip joint through its normal range of motion. Movements like lifting the knee or rotating the hip might be challenging.

- Muscle weakness or spasms around the hip joint can occur as the body's protective response to the injury, aiming to prevent further damage.

- Walking or putting weight on the affected leg might be uncomfortable or painful due to the strain on the injured ligaments.

- A sense or feeling of instability in the hip joint, as the ligaments' function in maintaining joint stability has been compromised.

Causes of Hip Sprain:

- Direct impact to the hip, whether from falling, colliding or close contact with another athlete during sports. This impact can stretch the ligaments beyond their usual range of motion.

- Rapid twisting or rotating actions of the hip joint can strain the ligaments. This occurs in sports which necessitates abrupt shifts in direction, pivoting, or twisting, mainly when the foot is planted and the body is in motion. It will occur in sports such as football, tennis and gymnastics.

- Overextending the hip joint past its natural range of motion, which occurs due to improper movements or excessive stretching.

- High-impact sports such as running, jumping, abrupt halts, and changes in direction increase the risk of hip joint sprains. Sports like soccer, basketball, and football involve such motions, increasing the likelihood of hip sprains.

- Weakness or imbalances in the muscles surrounding the hip joint can lead to instability, making the ligaments susceptible to injury during physical activities.

- Participating in activities involving repetitive motions, such as running, can gradually strain the ligaments encircling the hip joint over time. This can lead to sprain of the ligaments.

- Poor technique, like landing incorrectly after jumps or falls, can unevenly stress the hip joint, heightening its vulnerability to sprains.

Hip and Upper Leg Strains

Two of the most common injuries which occur at the hip and upper leg are the Hip Flexor Strain and Hamstring strain

A **hip flexor strain** is an injury that affects the muscles and tendons in the hip flexor region, located at the front of the hip. This group of muscles includes the iliopsoas, rectus femoris, tensor fasciae latae and sartorius (look at knee chapter). Hip flexors play a vital role in flexing the hip joint, which occurs when you bring your thigh towards your torso. This motion is involved in activities like walking, running, kicking, and lifting your legs.

Hip flexor strains occur when the above muscles and tendons are subjected to excessive force, stretching, or tearing. The severity of the strain can vary, leading to three different grades;

- **Grade 1:** This is a mild strain involving minimal stretching or microscopic tearing of muscle fibres. It may cause slight discomfort and might not significantly impact movement or function.

- **Grade 2:** A moderate strain characterized by more substantial tearing of muscle fibres. This grade can lead to moderate pain, reduced strength in hip flexion, and limitations in movement.

- **Grade 3:** A severe strain that involves a complete tear of the muscle or tendon. This is associated with significant pain, noticeable weakness, and difficulties in moving the leg.

Causes of Hip flexor strains include:

- Rapid or forceful movements that involve forcefully stretching the hip flexor muscles, such as sudden acceleration during sprinting or performing a forceful kick.
- Engaging in repetitive activities that strain the hip flexors, especially without adequate warm-up or conditioning.
- Weak hip flexor muscles or imbalances in muscle strength can make the area more susceptible to injury.
- Poor form during exercises or sports can increase the likelihood of straining the hip flexors.
- Muscles that are tight or not properly stretched (warming up) before engaging in activity can be more prone to strains.

Symptoms of a hip flexor strain include:

- Pain in the front of the hip or groin area.
- Discomfort when flexing the hip, especially during activities like lifting the knee or kicking.
- Swelling and bruising may occur in more severe cases.
- Restricted range of motion and difficulty performing actions like walking, running, or climbing stairs.
- Muscle spasms and tightness.

Tests for hip flexor strain:

- **Thomas Test**: This test assesses the flexibility of the hip flexors, particularly the iliopsoas muscle.[1] The patient lies on their back on an examination table and brings one knee towards the chest while keeping the other leg extended. If the extended leg lifts off the table, it indicates tightness in the hip flexors.

- **Ober's Test**: This test evaluates the tightness of the tensor fasciae latae (TFL) and iliotibial band (IT band).[2] The patient lies on their side with the lower leg flexed at the knee. The upper leg is abducted and then released it. If the leg remains elevated, it suggests tightness in the TFL and IT band.

- **Hip Flexor Strength Test**: This involves assessing the strength of the hip flexor muscles. The patient lies on their back with one leg extended and the other leg flexed at the hip and knee. They are asked to lift the extended leg off the table while the practitioner provides resistance. Weakness or pain during this movement might indicate a hip flexor strain.

- **Palpating the hip flexor muscles** and surrounding areas to identify areas of tenderness, swelling, or muscle tension.

Hamstring Strain

A hamstring strain, also known as a pulled hamstring, is an injury that occurs when the muscles or tendons at the back of the thigh are stretched or torn. A hamstring strain typically occurs during activities that involve explosive movements, sudden acceleration or deceleration, or excessive stretching of the hamstring muscles. Hamstring strains are common in sports that involve sprinting or sudden changes in direction, such as soccer, football, and track and field. They can also occur in activities that involve a sudden, forceful stretch of the hamstring muscles.

A hamstring strain primarily affects the hamstring muscles and their associated tendons. The muscles affected are the biceps femoris, semitendinosus and semimembranosus are located at the back of the thigh and are responsible for flexing the knee and extending the hip. When a strain occurs, it involves the stretching or tearing of muscle fibres and/or tendons. The severity can range from mild to severe. In severe cases, adjacent structures like blood vessels or nerves may also be affected.

Hamstring strains, both acute and chronic can be quite common in athletes and musculoskeletal injuries.

The severity of the strain can also be graded as with other strains, that is grade 1 being the mildest to grade 3 being the most severe.

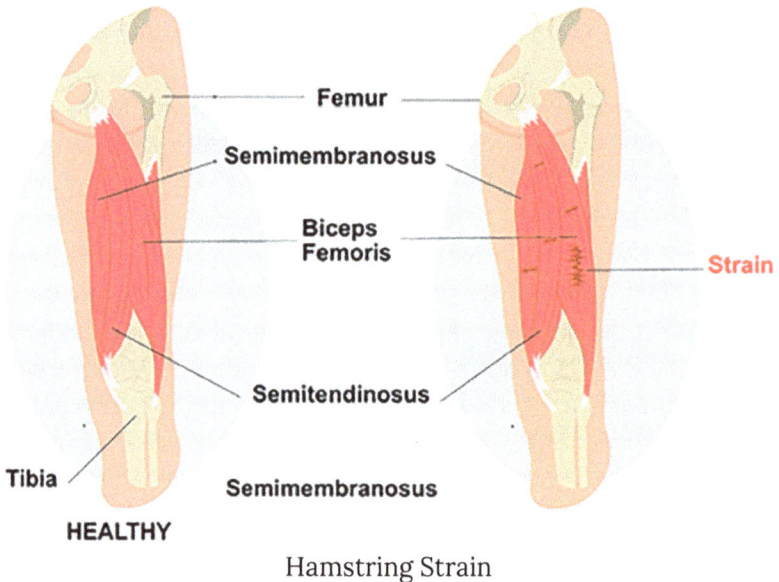

Femur
Semimembranosus
Biceps Femoris
Strain
Semitendinosus
Tibia
Semimembranosus
HEALTHY

Hamstring Strain

Causes of Hamstring Strains:

• Abrupt changes in speed or direction: Engaging in activities that involve sudden bursts of speed or abrupt stops, like sprinting or rapid changes in direction, can place significant strain on the hamstring muscles. This strain can occur if the muscles are not adequately prepared or conditioned.

- Excessive stretching: When the hamstring muscles are stretched beyond their usual range of motion, it can lead to tiny tears in the muscle fibres. This can happen during activities like stretching, kicking, or reaching for an object while extending the leg.

- Failure to warm up adequately: Neglecting to properly warm up before engaging in strenuous physical activity can heighten the risk of a hamstring strain. Muscles that are cold and tight are more prone to injury, so it's crucial to gradually warm up to increase blood flow and flexibility.

- Muscle fatigue: Fatigued muscles are more vulnerable to strains. When muscles are tired, they might not be able to absorb and disperse force effectively, making them more susceptible to becoming overstressed.

- Previous injury: If there has been a prior hamstring strain that hasn't fully healed or wasn't properly rehabilitated, the area may be weaker and more prone to re-injury.

- Improper technique: Using incorrect form or technique during physical activities can add extra stress to the hamstring muscles, increasing the risk of a strain.

- Inadequate flexibility or strength: If the hamstring muscles are not sufficiently conditioned or if there's an imbalance in strength between the hamstrings and other leg muscles, it can heighten the risk of a strain.

- Age-related: As individuals age, their muscles tend to lose some flexibility and elasticity, making them more susceptible to strains.

- Sudden force or impact: Direct trauma or force applied to the back of the thigh, such as from a fall or collision, can lead to a hamstring strain.

- Tightness or imbalance in other muscles: Muscles that oppose the action of the hamstrings (such as the quadriceps at the front of the thigh) can contribute to strain if they are significantly stronger or tighter.

- Insufficient rehabilitation: Failing to adequately rehabilitate a prior hamstring injury can result in ongoing weakness and a greater vulnerability to re-injury.

Symptoms of Hamstring Strains:

- Pain: The pain associated with a hamstring strain is typically felt in the back of the thigh, and it can range from a mild ache to a sharp, severe pain. The pain is often aggravated by activities that engage the hamstring muscles, such as walking, running, or bending the knee.

- Tenderness: Upon touching or pressing the affected area, there may be tenderness. This tenderness is localized to the back of the thigh where the strain has occurred.

- Swelling: Depending on the severity of the strain, there may be varying degrees of swelling around the injured area. In more severe cases, significant swelling can be observed.

- Bruising or ecchymosis: In cases of more significant strains, bleeding within the muscle tissue can lead to the development of bruising. This can result in discoloration of the skin around the injured area.

- Weakness: The affected leg may feel weaker than the uninjured leg. This weakness is particularly noticeable when attempting to engage the hamstring muscles, such as when trying to bend the knee or extend the hip against resistance.

- Difficulty walking: Depending on the severity of the strain, walking can be challenging. In severe cases, it may be nearly impossible to bear weight on the affected leg, leading to a limp or altered gait.

- Limited range of motion: Movements that involve bending the knee or extending the hip may be restricted or painful.

Fully extending the leg or bending the knee against resistance may be especially difficult.

- Muscle spasms: As a protective mechanism, the injured muscle may go into spasms. These involuntary contractions can be painful and may contribute to the overall discomfort experienced.

- Popping or snapping sensation: Some patients may report feeling or even hearing a popping or snapping sensation at the time of injury. This can be indicative of a tear or rupture within the muscle fibres.

- Stiffness: After a period of inactivity, such as after sleeping or sitting for an extended period, the hamstring area may feel stiff and require a bit of time and movement to loosen up.

Labral Tears

The labrum, a cartilage ring that surrounds the acetabulum functions as a cushion and stabilizer for the hip joint, enhancing its functionality and providing support during movements at the hip.

Several factors can contribute to the development of labral tears:

- A direct impact to the hip, like a fall or collision, can result in labral tearing or damage. Such incidents lead to sudden, acute injuries often accompanied by intense pain.

- Activities involving frequent hip movement, pivoting, and rotation which are common in sports like soccer, hockey, or dance. There is a gradual wearing down or tear of the labrum due to continuous stress.

- Hip impingement, also known as femoroacetabular impingement (FAI), is a condition where there is abnormal contact between the femoral head and acetabulum of the hip joint. This can occur due to structural abnormalities in the hip bones that result in an improper fit between these two surfaces. The friction and repetitive contact caused by hip impingement can lead to pain, cartilage damage, and labral tears over time.

- Improper development of the hip joint, known as Hip Dysplasia, can lead to instability and misalignment, putting the labrum at risk of damage due to unusual stress.

- With age, the labrum can undergo degenerative changes, becoming thinner and more vulnerable to injury. This is more common among older adults and can contribute to labral tears.

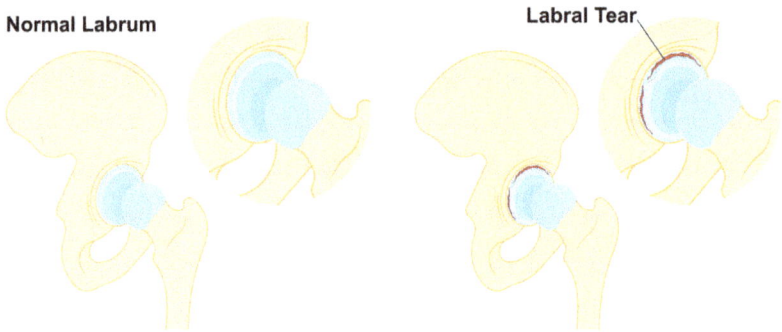

Normal Labrum

Labral Tear

Hip Labral Tears

Symptoms of a hip labral injury include:

- Hip pain or groin discomfort may be felt as a deep ache or pulsating sensation, is the most significant presenting symptom. Although this is often localized in the groin region, it potentially extends to the buttocks or anterior thigh.

- Sensation of clicking or "catching" may be present in some patients. This sensation of clicking, catching, or even popping is felt within the hip joint during certain movements.

- Restricted range of motion with joint stiffness and diminished flexibility, resulting in a constrained range of motion. Everyday activities such as hip flexion, rotation, or leg crossing may exhibit reduced capacity.

- Discomfort during prolonged sitting or standing may increase particularly on hard surfaces.

- Instability or muscular weakness.

- When the labrum injury is mild, participating in sports or activities that necessitate rapid changes in direction, pivoting, or high-impact movements can exacerbate the pain associated with a labral injury.

Labral injuries can sometimes be confused with other hip-related conditions such as hip flexor strains or osteoarthritis. Several tests such as the FABER and FADIR tests can be performed to indicate labral injuries. However, carrying out these tests requires experience and skill. Imaging such as MRA, ultrasound, x-ray and c-scan are most revealing of labral injuries. Note x-rays do not directly show labral tears, but they can help identify any bony abnormalities, such as femoroacetabular impingement, which can contribute to labral tears.

FABER test is testing for flexion, abduction and external rotation and involves moving the hip joint through a combination of flexion, abduction, and external rotation to evaluate any pain or discomfort, which can indicate labral issues.

FADIR test is flexion, adduction and internal rotation to assess pain and discomfort in the hip during flexion, adduction, and internal rotation, potentially indicating labral tears.

Bursitis

Bursitis is a painful condition that occurs when the bursae, small fluid-filled sacs located near joints, become inflamed.

Bursae act as cushions between bones, tendons, muscles, and skin, reducing friction during movement. There are a number of bursae around the hip, however two bursae usually affected are;

i) Trochanteric Bursa: Located on the outer part of the hip, covering the greater trochanter.

ii) Iliopsoas Bursa: This bursa is located on the inside of the hip, deep in the pelvis. It lies between the iliopsoas tendon (a hip flexor muscle) and the underlying bone.

Hip bursitis commonly affects the trochanteric bursitis, and less frequently, the iliopsoas bursa on the inside the hip joint. Upper thigh bursitis can also include the ischial bursa, which is near the ischial tuberosities. Ischial bursitis can result from prolonged sitting on hard surfaces or direct trauma.

Hip bursitis is often caused by repetitive activities like running or cycling, muscle imbalances, or tightness. Hip bursitis can occur in sports due to repetitive movements, overuse, or direct trauma to the hip region. Sports that involve frequent hip movements, running, jumping, or sudden changes in direction can increase the risk of developing hip bursitis.

Symptoms include pain, tenderness, swelling, restricted range of motion, and discomfort during activities involving the affected area.

Athletic Pubalgia

Also known as sports hernia, is a condition characterized by chronic groin pain in athletes.[3] It is not a typical hernia with a visible bulge, but rather an injury to the soft tissues in the lower abdomen and groin area. Athletic Pubalgia often arises from repetitive stress in sports involving sudden movements and forceful contractions. Symptoms include persistent and chronic groin pain, tenderness, and pain during exercise. Unlike a typical hernia, there is usually no visible bulge or protrusion in the skin. Diagnosis of the condition is difficult and usually requires use of ultrasound and MRI imaging.

Athletic Pubalgia primarily affects the soft tissues in the lower abdomen and groin area. The anatomical structures that are commonly affected in Athletic Pubalgia include:

- Rectus Abdominis Muscle: This is one of the main muscles of the abdomen, running vertically from the lower part of the ribcage down to the pubic bone.

- Adductor Muscles: These muscles are located on the inner thigh and are responsible for bringing the legs together.

- Inguinal Ligament: This is a band of connective tissue that runs from the pubic bone to the anterior superior iliac spine, forming the lower border of the abdomen.

- Pectineus Muscle: This is a small muscle located in the groin area, responsible for adducting and flexing the hip.

- Pubic Symphysis: Ligaments and cartilage around the two pubic bones where they meet at the front of the pelvis.

- Transversalis Fascia: This is a layer of connective tissue that lines the inside of the abdominal wall.

TCM Treatment of the HIP and Upper Leg Injuries

In Traditional Chinese Medicine, the understanding of pathological conditions centres around the disharmony in the flow of Qi and Blood along the body's meridians, as well as the disruption in the equilibrium between Yin and Yang. These imbalances manifest as various syndrome patterns.

While Western Medical knowledge explains and treats specific issues such as labral tears, hip flexor strains and sprains, TCM interprets these conditions as physical conditions as well as patterns of disharmony. Acupuncture points are carefully chosen for their capacity to restore balance to these disharmonies.

Acupuncture can offer benefits for acute hip injuries by helping to alleviate pain, inflammation, and muscle tension. However, during this phase, it is **vital to avoid** needling directly into areas with acute inflammation, bruising, or open wounds. Needling an acutely injured area can exacerbate the inflammatory response and so be more harmful. During this phase, it is better to use adjacent, distal, corresponding or auricular points all of which should be approached with gentle needling. During acute phase, PRICE; Protect, Rest, Ice, Compression and Elevation will dampen the presenting inflammation.

As injuries transition from the acute to subacute phase acupuncture can support the body's natural healing mechanisms and the aim of the treatment is to relieve pain, clear heat, resolve toxins and dispel local stasis.

With chronic injuries acupuncture will enhance circulation, and facilitate healing. Treatment focus may shift towards addressing underlying imbalances contributing to long-standing issues such as organ pathology

Local and Adjacent points for Hip and Thigh Pain

Please see Appendix 1 for Acupuncture Point Location.

- **GB30** is an essential point for hip disorders as its use promotes Qi and Blood, activates the channel, alleviates pain, and is helpful for both Qi and Blood stagnation. The point benefits the hip. When the pain radiates to the upper leg and if lumbar region is painful combine GB30 with BL40.

- GB30 is also useful point to use for trochanteric bursa (both acute and chronic) and partial labral tears.
- When the knee is affected, combine with ST33 and ST40.
- If the groin is painful, combine with GB29 and LIV9.

Needling: 1.5cun – 2.5cun, needled towards the groin, patient in the lateral recumbent position, and thigh flexed.

- **GB29** is a commonly used point to treat hip disorders, mainly when the pain radiates to the groin area, such as sports hernia. Can be used with GB20 as this relaxes the sinews and invigorates channels (softens muscles).

Also, useful when pain radiates to the thigh area, when pain may be due to trochanteric bursitis and labral tears.

Needling: perpendicular 2cun to 3cun

- **ST31** activates the channel and alleviates pain. Point is used when the hip and the anterior thigh muscles are symptomatic with symptoms of pain and stiffness. Also, useful if there is an accompanying weakness of the knee. As part of the lower kinetic chain, the knee can be affected when the hip is injured (as the knee may try to compensate for the hip). Combine with ST36 and ST41. This combination of points is useful where the anterior group of muscles are affected such as in hip flexor strains.

ST31 also regulates the circulation of Qi and Blood in the whole limb (stomach Yang Ming is rich in Blood and Qi) and warming the channel, so it can be used in cold obstruction syndrome.

Needling: perpendicular 1cun to 2cun

- **ST32** is another point which can be used for anterior thigh pain and stiffness, specifically when the rectus femoris is affected (part of the quadriceps). A useful point to use when the quadriceps muscles are strained, the knee is painful, or there is weakness. Rectus femoris is the only muscle of the quadriceps to cross both the hip and knee joints, flexing the thigh and extending the knee (hence injury to the muscle also affects the knee joint)

Needling: perpendicular 1cun to 2cun

- **BL36** activates the bladder channel, alleviates pain, and relaxes the sinews. These characteristics make it ideal for hamstring tendinopathies (both acute and chronic). A useful point when pain is referred to the gluteal region, with sciatica, or when pain and stiffness are felt along the bladder channel.

  Needling: perpendicular 1cun to 2cun

Other Less Commonly Used Points:

- **GB31:** Used for thigh pain and weakness.

- **UB32:** Used in conjunction with UB31 for hip and sacroiliac pain.

- **UB40:** used for addressing pain and tension in the thigh and hip area. Also useful for pain in lumbar area.

- **SP10:** Used for various conditions affecting the lower extremities, including hip and thigh pain.

The channels affected by hip injury are:

- Anterior thigh: Stomach, Liver and Spleen channels

- Posterior thigh: Urinary Bladder channel.

- Lateral aspect: Gall Bladder channel.

- Medial aspect: Spleen channel.

Distal Points for Hip and Thigh Pain

- **BL60:** Activates the bladder channel and alleviates pain along the bladder channel, including the lumbar, sacral and posterior aspect of the knee and distally the ankle. If the lumbar region is also symptomatic (with a hip injury), combine with GB30 and BL40. Relaxes the sinews. Useful for hamstring tendinopathy.

  Needling: perpendicular 0.5cun to 1cun. Caution, contraindicated in pregnancy.

- **BL62** relaxes sinews and alleviates pain, especially when pain is felt along the bladder channel. Opens and regulates Yang Motility channels.

  Needling: perpendicular 0.3cun to 0.5cun

- **BL40** is a useful point to use when the athlete has hip and severe lumbar pain and stiffness. Activates the channel and so alleviates pain. BL 40 can also be used for recurring symptoms.

  Needling: perpendicular (but at a slight angle, otherwise the flow of Qi interrupted) 1.0cun to 1.5cun

Other useful points and combinations for hip and thigh:

- GB29, GB30, BL54, and ST31 can be used locally to promote the circulation of Qi and Blood (in channels and collaterals) to remove stagnation and relieve pain.

- If pain or symptoms are felt along the Bladder channel, the hamstrings, BL36, BL58, and BL63, can be used. These points harmonize collaterals and relieve pain.

- If pain or symptoms are felt along the Gall Bladder channel (lateral aspect of the thigh), GB34, GB36, and GB40 to promote Qi and Blood and relieve pain.

- If pain or symptoms are felt along the Stomach channel, that is, the quadriceps group of muscles, ST30, ST34, ST40, and ST42 can be used as these promote the circulation of Qi and Blood (stagnation) and relieve pain.

Constitutional Supporting Points

GB34: Found on the outer leg below the knee, this point is often used to relieve pain and inflammation in the hip joint.

SP6: Situated on the inner leg above the ankle, SP6 is known for its ability to harmonize and balance the body's energy, potentially aiding hip-related imbalances.

LI4: Located on the hand, LI4 has a pain-relieving effect that could benefit hip discomfort.

ST36: Positioned on the lower leg, ST36 is thought to boost overall Qi and circulation, potentially aiding in healing.

LIV3: Found on the foot, LIV3 is often used for pain relief and promoting the smooth flow of Qi.

Auricular points

The systemic auricular points for hip pain are: Shen men, Thalamus, Adrenal, Endocrine as well as the hip point.

Corresponding points, Hip/Shoulder

BL36 to SI10, GB30 to SJ14, ST30 to LI15, SP12 to LU2 and LIV12 to PC2

Hip Bi Syndrome

Bi Syndrome is caused by external pathogenic factors, Cold, Damp, Heat and Wind, collectively known as Xie. When the pathogenic factors invade the body, these Xie disrupt the body's balance and energy flow, leading to symptoms like pain and stiffness. Additionally, if the body's protective energy, Wei Qi, is weak, it can't effectively repel Xie, allowing them to penetrate deeper and worsen the condition. With hip, common patterns of Bi and its treatment are explained below.

Common Bi Syndrome Patterns of the Hip:

- *Wind-Cold Bi Syndrome*: This type of Bi syndrome involves the invasion of Wind and Cold Xie into the hip joint. It leads to sudden and shifting pain, stiffness, and a feeling of coldness in the affected area. The pain might worsen in cold weather and improve with warmth.

  GB30: Helps dispel Wind and Cold, promoting circulation and relieving pain.

  GB31: Can help relieve hip pain, particularly when caused by Wind-Cold Bi.

- *Wind-Damp Bi Syndrome*: Wind and Dampness are combined Xie that invade the hip joint. This can cause a sensation of heaviness, swelling, and aching pain. The pain tends to be more pronounced during damp and humid weather.

  GB34: Expels Dampness and promotes Qi flow to alleviate pain.

  SP9: Helps to resolve Dampness and promotes circulation.

- *Cold-Damp Bi Syndrome*: Cold and Damp Xie combine to cause pain that is both cold and damp in nature. The hip may feel heavy, stiff, and swollen, with pain that worsens in cold and damp conditions.

  SP6: Helps to regulate Dampness and harmonize the Spleen.

  UB23: Warms the Kidneys and dispels Cold.

- *Heat Bi Syndrome*: Heat Xie can also affect the hip, causing symptoms like redness, swelling, and intense pain. The pain might feel hot and sharp, and the area might be warm to the touch.

  LI11: Clears Heat and reduces inflammation.

  SP10: Cools Heat and reduces excessive Fire.

- *Phlegm-Damp Bi Syndrome*: Phlegm and Dampness Xie can contribute to a feeling of heaviness, stiffness, and numbness in the hip area. The pain might be dull and persistent, and there could be a sense of swelling or puffiness.

  ST40: Resolves Dampness and Phlegm in the body.

  SP9: Resolves Dampness and harmonizes the Spleen.

Conclusion

Acupuncture is valuable in treating hip and upper leg injuries which are quite common in sports and musculoskeletal injuries. By enhancing Qi and Blood flow to the affected area, acupuncture triggers the body's innate healing responses, leading to recovery of damaged tissues. By focussing on specific acupuncture points, treatment also helps to relax tense muscles and alleviate spasms and so improving flexibility and range of motion.

References

1. www:physiotutors.com/wiki/thomas-test/.
2. www:physio-pedia.com/Ober Test.
3. www:orthoinfo.aaos.org/en/diseases-conditions/sports-hernia-athletic-pubalgia.

Chapter 15

Part 1 – Knee Anatomy

The knee joint plays an important role in sports activities by enabling a range of movements and actions. Its primary functions include providing stability for balance and control, bearing a substantial portion of the body's weight, and facilitating essential motions such as flexion and extension. The joint also serves as a shock absorber during high-impact actions like jumping and landing, protecting against injuries. The knee joint is a synovial, hinge joint that connects the femur, tibia, and patella.[1] The knee joint, primarily allows flexion of 140 degrees and extension of 0 degrees. It also allows rotational movement and medial and lateral glide when the knee is partially bent.

Knee Joint

The femur, the body's longest and strongest bone, forms the upper part of the knee joint. Its rounded condyles at the distal end articulate with the proximal part of the tibia. The tibia constitutes the more prominent lower leg bone and complements the knee joint's structure. It supports body weight and facilitates force transmission from the femur to the foot.

The patella, a small, triangular bone, is positioned in front of the knee joint and is enclosed within the quadriceps tendon. The patella enhances the mechanical advantage of the powerful quadriceps muscles during leg extension.

Inside the knee joint, two crescent-shaped fibrocartilaginous structures known as menisci lie between the femoral condyles and the tibial plateau. The menisci act as shock absorbers, distributing weight and forces evenly to protect the joint from excessive wear. The synovium, a thin, smooth membrane, lines the inner surface of the knee joint. It produces synovial fluid, a lubricating substance that nourishes the joint and reduces bone friction, facilitating smooth movements.

Knee Joint Capsule

The knee joint capsule is a complex structure that encircles the knee joint, making the joint stable and preventing excessive movement. It consists of two primary layers, an outer fibrous layer and an inner synovial membrane.

The outer fibrous layer is the external part of the knee joint capsule comprising of sturdy and dense fibrous connective tissue. Its role is to uphold the knee joint's structural integrity, protecting it from external pressures and potential injuries. The layer, firmly attaches to the bones of the knee joint, including the femur and tibia. It also links with the menisci and nearby ligaments, providing to the knee joint's stability.

The internal layer of the knee joint capsule is the synovial membrane, is thinner and less dense than the outer fibrous layer. This membrane lines the interior of the joint capsule and functions to provide synovial fluid which provides lubrication and is a source of nutrients within the joint cavity.

Knee Joint Ligaments

The knee joint relies on several ligaments to maintain stability and prevent excessive movement. These internal ligaments include:

- **Anterior Cruciate Ligament (ACL):** Running diagonally inside the knee, the ACL connects the front of the tibia to the back of the femur. Its role is to stop the femur from sliding forward on the tibia and provide rotational stability, especially during activities that involve sudden changes in direction.

- **Posterior Cruciate Ligament (PCL):** Also, diagonal but opposite to the ACL, the PCL connects the back of the tibia to the front of the femur. It prevents the femur from sliding backwards on the tibia and provides rotational stability, especially when bending the knee with weight-bearing actions.

- **Medial Collateral Ligament (MCL):** Situated on the inner side of the knee, the MCL connects the inner part of the femur to the medial side of the tibia. It offers stability against inward forces that may impact the knee from the lateral side.

- **Lateral Collateral Ligament (LCL):** Found on the outer side of the knee, the LCL connects the outer part of the femur to the lateral side of the tibia. It provides stability against outward forces that may impact the knee, mirroring the function of the MCL but on the opposite side.

The above ligaments work together to stabilize the knee joint and are important for joint integrity and reducing injury risks associated with weight-bearing and dynamic movements.

In addition to the four main ligaments above, there are other ligaments present at the knee joint, providing extra stability and support:

- **Oblique Popliteal Ligament:** Extending from the semimembranosus tendon (a hamstring muscle), the ligament reinforces the back of the knee joint and helps

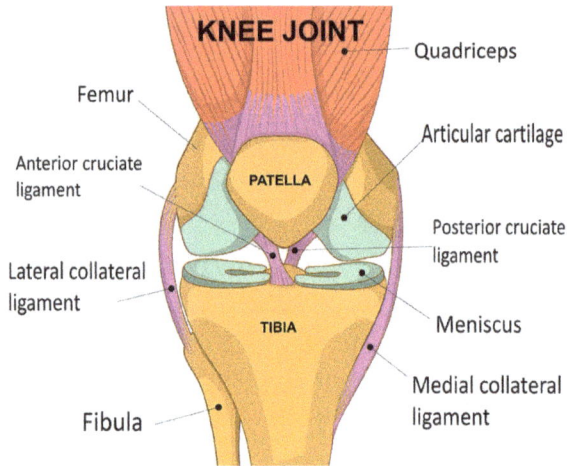

KNEE JOINT

Quadriceps

Femur

Articular cartilage

Anterior cruciate ligament

PATELLA

Posterior cruciate ligament

Lateral collateral ligament

TIBIA

Meniscus

Medial collateral ligament

Fibula

Knee Joint

to prevent excessive hyperextension of the knee. It blends with the posterior knee capsule, offering additional support and stability.

- **The Patellar Ligament:** Also known as the patellar tendon (as it connects a muscle to a bone), extends the quadriceps muscles to the tibia, facilitating knee extension during activities like jumping and running. The patellar ligament's function is to transmit forces generated by the quadriceps muscles to the lower leg during weight-bearing activities. It also assists in stabilizing the patella within the patellar groove on the front of the femur. Injuries to the patellar ligament, such as patellar tendonitis (also known as jumper's knee) or complete tears, can impact an athlete's ability to extend the knee and participate in various activities.

Muscles Acting on the Knee Joint

The main movement at the knee is *flexion* and *extension*. The primary group of muscles functioning as knee flexors are the hamstrings, while the muscles extending the knee are the quadriceps.

• Knee Extensors – The Quadriceps Femoris Group

This is a group of four muscles, the Rectus Femoris, Vastus Lateralis, Vastus Medialis, and Vastus Intermedius, located on the anterior aspect of the thigh.[2] The three vastus muscles originate from the femur, while the rectus femoris originates from the anterior inferior iliac spine. The quadriceps muscles converge to form the quadriceps tendon, which surrounds and encases the patella. The quadriceps tendon then continues as the patellar ligament to attach to the tibial tuberosity. This allows the quadriceps muscles to work collectively to extend the knee joint and facilitate movements involving the lower limb. Contributes to activities such as jumping, sprinting, kicking, and squatting. They enable explosive power and stability when extending the leg.

• Knee Flexors – The Hamstrings

The hamstring muscles include the biceps femoris, semitendinosus, and semimembranosus. These muscles are located on the posterior aspect of the thigh (back) and act as knee flexors.[3] The hamstrings muscles are responsible for flexing the knee joint and extending the hip joint, allowing activities like bending over, sitting down, and performing leg curls.

- **Biceps Femoris:** Long head originates from the ischial tuberosity of the pelvis. The short head originates from the lateral lip of the linea aspera of the femur. Both heads merge and attach to the head of the fibula, a lower leg bone.

- **Semitendinosus:** Also originates from the ischial tuberosity of the pelvis and inserts into the medial surface of the upper part of the tibia, just below the tibial plateau.

- **Semimembranosus:** Originates from Ischial tuberosity of the pelvis and inserts into the posterior surface of the medial condyle of the tibia, just below the semitendinosus attachment.

TENDONS OF THE KNEE

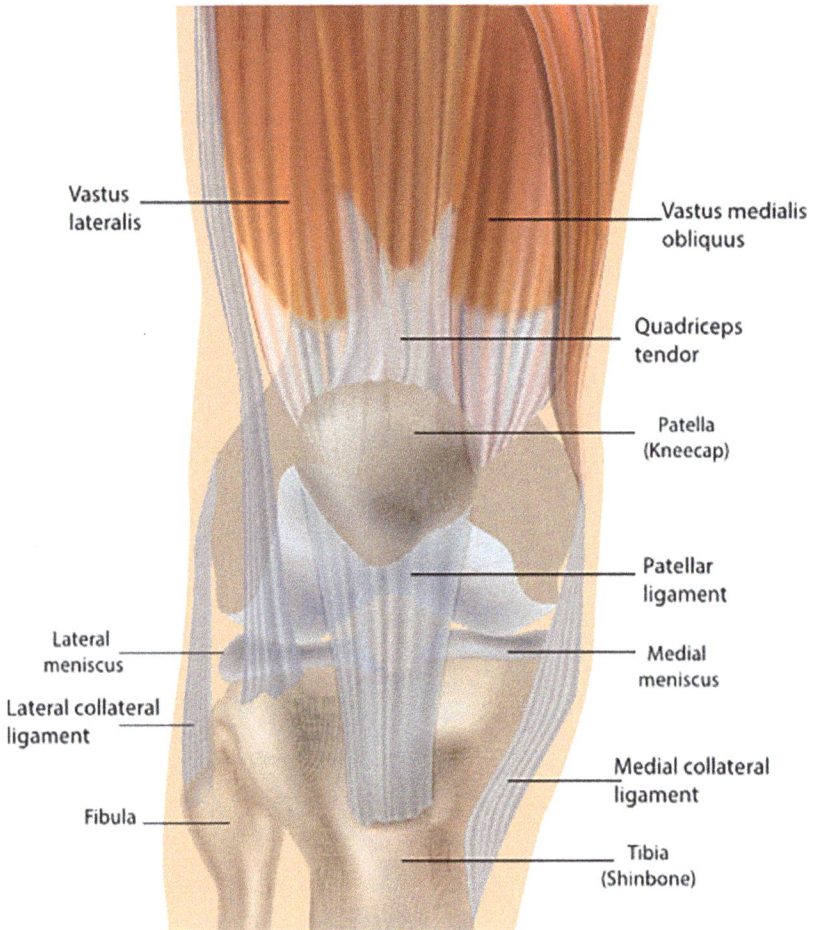

Vastus lateralis

Vastus medialis obliquus

Quadriceps tendor

Patella (Kneecap)

Patellar ligament

Lateral meniscus

Medial meniscus

Lateral collateral ligament

Medial collateral ligament

Fibula

Tibia (Shinbone)

Knee tendons

In sports, injuries to the hamstrings can be relatively common, particularly in sports that involve sprinting, jumping, and sudden changes in speed and direction. The hamstrings play a part in both acceleration and deceleration movements.

• Popliteus Muscle

The Popliteus muscle is a small but important muscle behind the knee joint. It originates from the lateral condyle of the femur and inserts into the upper part of the tibia. Its primary function is to unlock the knee joint by initiating knee flexion and assisting in the inward rotation of the tibia.[4] This action is vital for smooth and controlled knee bending during pivoting and cutting movements in sports such as basketball, soccer, and tennis. The popliteus muscle prevents knee injuries and ensures efficient movements during athletic activities.

Conclusion

The knee which is a complex hinge joint plays an essential role in sports activities and performance for weight-bearing and locomotion. Its anatomy involves bones, ligaments, tendons, and cartilage all functioning in synchronisation. The femur, tibia, and patella form the joint's foundation, while ligaments provide stability, and menisci cushion and distribute forces. Muscles surrounding the knee, particularly the quadriceps and hamstrings, play an essential role in movement and stabilization. Common disorders, such as ligament injuries, meniscal tears, and osteoarthritis, can significantly impact an athlete's performance and also affect the patient's overall quality of life. Understanding the structure of the knee is essential for comprehending its function and for diagnosing and treating injuries or conditions affecting this vital joint.

References

1. www:kenhub.com/en/study/anatomy-knee-joint.
2. www:physio-pedia.com/QuadricepsMuscle.
3. www:orthoinfo.aaos.org/en/diseases--conditions/hamstring-muscle-injuries.
4. www:kenhub.com/en/library/anatomy/popliteus-muscle.

Chapter 15

Part 2 – Knee & Lower Leg Injuries and TCM Treatment

Sports and musculoskeletal injuries of the knee are a persistent challenge in athletes when participating in sports and physical activities. As a pivotal hinge joint, the knee plays a central role in an athlete's ability to perform a wide range of movements, from running and jumping to cutting and pivoting. However, the very demands of these actions can subject the knee to significant stresses and strains, making it susceptible to various injuries. Understanding the complexities of knee anatomy and how this may relate to specific mechanisms underlying these injuries is essential for accurate diagnosis, effective treatment, and, also for the development of preventative strategies.

Knee Sprain

A knee sprain can affect various ligaments within the knee, and the specific ligaments involved will determine the type of knee sprain and the associated symptoms. The main ligaments that can be affected by a knee sprain are;

Anterior Cruciate Ligament (ACL)

The ACL runs diagonally in the middle of the knee, connecting the femur to the tibia. ACL sprains are common sports injuries. Symptoms of an ACL sprain may include a sudden, audible "pop" at the time of injury, followed by:

- Rapid and severe swelling.
- A feeling of instability or the knee giving way.
- Difficulty bearing weight on the injured leg.
- Pain and tenderness along the joint line.
- Limited range of motion.
- Feeling of joint laxity or looseness.

The Lachman test and the anterior drawer test are used to assess the ACL.[1] During this test, the patient's knee is slightly bent, and the examiner gently applies an anterior force to the lower leg while stabilizing the thigh. The key observation is any excess forward movement of the tibia and the presence of a soft feeling in the knee. A positive result is indicative of an ACL injury.

Posterior Cruciate Ligament (PCL)

The PCL is another ligament within the knee, but it is less commonly injured than the ACL. The posterior cruciate ligament connects the femur to the tibia inside the knee joint. It prevents the shin bone from moving too far backward in relation to the thigh bone. This ligament provides stability during activities like pivoting and cutting.

Symptoms of a PCL sprain may include:

- Swelling and pain at the back of the knee.
- A feeling of instability, especially when trying to move the knee.
- Pain and discomfort, particularly when trying to bend the knee.
- Difficulty walking or running.
- A sensation of the knee "giving way" during movements.

The *posterior drawer* test is a clinical assessment to evaluate the posterior cruciate ligament in the knee joint, primarily for PCL tears or sprains. During this test, the patient's knee is flexed at a 90-degree angle, and the examiner gently applies a backward force to the tibia while stabilizing the calf. The examination aims to detect excessive backward movement of the tibia and the presence of a soft or "mushy" feeling in the knee. A positive result suggests a potential PCL injury,

Medial Collateral Ligament (MCL)

The MCL is located on the medial aspect of the knee and helps stabilize the knee. Symptoms of an MCL sprain may include:

- Pain and tenderness along the inner side of the knee.
- Swelling in the area.
- A feeling of instability, particularly when the knee is bent sideways.
- Pain with activities that involve side-to-side movements.
- Mild to moderate joint laxity.

Lateral Collateral Ligament (LCL)

Situated on the lateral aspect of the knee, LCL sprains are less common than MCL sprains.

Symptoms of an LCL sprain may include:

- Pain and tenderness along the outer side of the knee.
- Swelling in the area.
- Instability or a feeling of giving way during movements.
- Pain with activities that put stress on the outer side of the knee.

Valgus and Varus stress tests are clinical examinations used to assess the MCL (medial collateral ligament) and LCL (lateral collateral ligament) in the knee, respectively.[2] In the valgus stress test for the MCL, the patient's knee is slightly bent, and the examiner applies an inward force, observing for excessive medial movement. In the varus stress test for LCL, an outward force is applied to the knee, and the examiner feels for excessive lateral movement. Positive results, indicating excessive movement or a "soft" feeling, may suggest ligament injury.

Patellofemoral Pain Syndrome (PFPS)

Also known as "runner's knee" or "anterior knee pain," is a knee condition characterized by pain and discomfort around the front of the knee where the patella and femur articulate. It arises due to improper tracking of the patella over the femoral groove during knee movement. Patella tracking is the alignment and movement of the patella within the groove at the front of the femur, the femoral groove.

Anatomical structures affected by Patellofemoral Pain Syndrome are Patella, the femur and the quadriceps muscles.

The exact cause of PFPS is not clear, but it is associated with the risk factors such as;

- Overuse or repetitive stress on the knee joint which may occur in activities like running, jumping, or squatting.

- Muscle imbalances or weakness, particularly in the quadriceps or hip muscles, lead to altered patellar tracking.

- Abnormalities in the knee joint or leg alignment include flat feet or increased "Q" angle. The "Q" angle is the angle created by the line connecting the anterior superior iliac spine to the middle of the patella and the line connecting the tibial tuberosity to the middle of the patella.

- Poor biomechanics or improper form during physical activities.
- Tightness or imbalance in the muscles and tendons around the knee joint.

Symptoms of Patellofemoral Pain Syndrome:

- Pain around the kneecap or behind the kneecap, particularly during activities that involve knee bending, such as walking, running, squatting, or stair climbing.
- The pain tends to worsen with physical activities and may ease during rest. In severe cases, pain can persist even during periods of inactivity.
- Some individuals with PFPS may experience a grinding or popping sensation during knee flexion and extension.
- Stiffness and reduced flexibility.
- Swelling and tenderness.
- Instability or a feeling of the knee giving way.

Knee Tendinitis

Also known as patellar tendinitis or jumper's knee, is when the patellar tendon around the knee joint becomes inflamed or irritated due to overuse. The patellar tendon connects the quadriceps muscles to the tibia and is crucial for knee extension and supporting high-impact activities like jumping and running. Knee tendinitis is more common among individuals who participate in sports or physical activities and those between the ages of 15 and 30.[3]

Causes and Risk Factors Associated with Knee Tendinitis:

- Repetitive overuse or excessive strain on the patellar tendon.

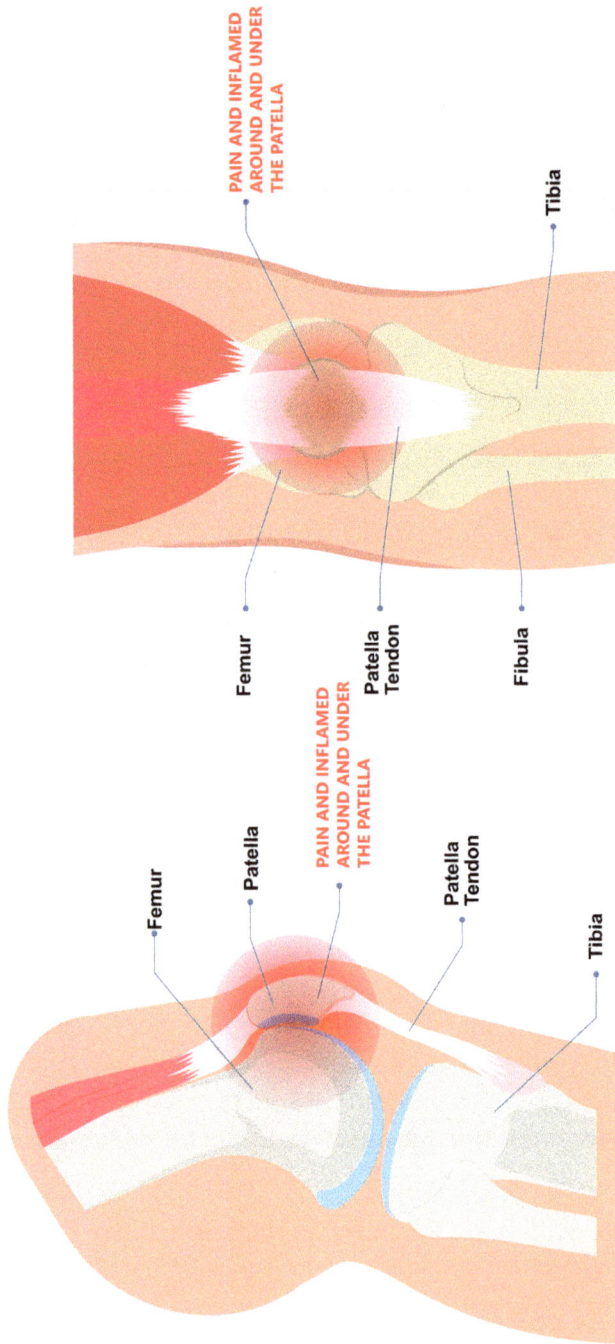

Patellofemoral Syndrome

PAIN AND INFLAMED AROUND AND UNDER THE PATELLA

Femur

Patella Tendon

Fibula

Tibia

Femur

Patella

PAIN AND INFLAMED AROUND AND UNDER THE PATELLA

Patella Tendon

Tibia

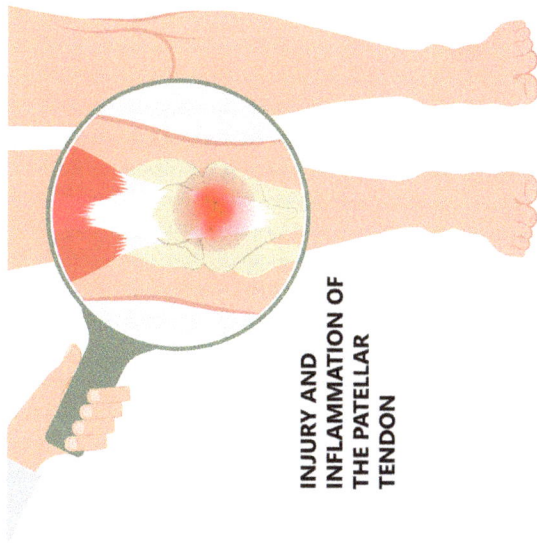

PATELLAR TENDONITIS - JUMPER'S KNEE

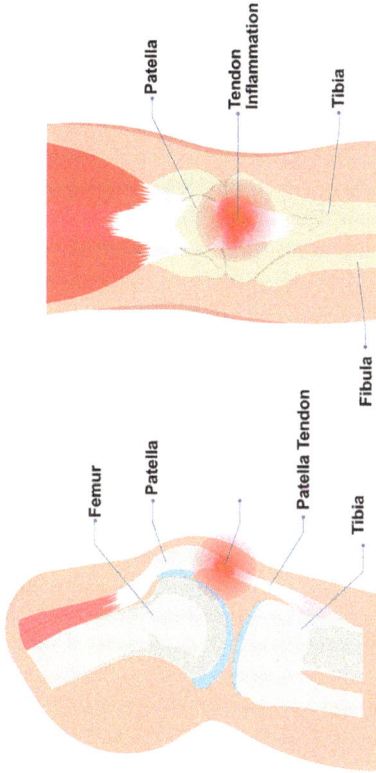

INJURY AND
INFLAMMATION OF
THE PATELLAR
TENDON

Patellar Tendinitis

- Engaging in sports or exercises that involve frequent jumping, running, or sudden changes in direction can strain the patellar tendon.

- Sudden increases in training intensity, inadequate warm-up, or improper technique during physical activities can lead to tendon irritation.

- Weakness or imbalances in the quadriceps muscles can increase stress on the patellar tendon.

- Poor Biomechanics and abnormalities in the knee or lower limb alignment, such as flat feet or patella misalignment, can contribute to tendon irritation.

- Past knee injuries, such as sprains or strains, can make the patellar tendon more susceptible to inflammation.

Symptoms below of knee tendinitis can vary in intensity and usually develop gradually:

- Anterior knee pain: The primary symptom is pain felt at the front of the knee, just below the patella.

- Pain during activity: The pain tends to worsen during activities that stress the patellar tendon, such as jumping, running, squatting, or climbing stairs.

- Morning stiffness: Some individuals may experience mild stiffness and discomfort in the knee upon waking or after rest.

- Tenderness and swelling: The area around the patellar tendon may feel tender to the touch, and there might be mild swelling.

- Quadriceps weakness: As the condition progresses, weakness in the quadriceps muscles can become noticeable.

- Crepitus: Some individuals might hear or feel a crackling sensation when moving the knee.

Iliotibial Band Syndrome (ITBS)

The iliotibial band (IT band) is a tough, fibrous band of connective tissue located on the outer side of the thigh. The IT band extends downward, running along the lateral part of the thigh and attaching to the tibia, just below the knee joint. Along its course, the IT band passes over the greater trochanter, of the femur. Its function is to stabilize the hip and knee joints during movement. The IT band originates from two main muscles, the tensor fasciae latae muscle located at the front of the hip and the gluteus maximus muscle of the buttocks. The IT band interacts with various muscles around the hip and thigh, including the glutes, quadriceps, and hamstrings, contributing to coordinated movement. ITBS occurs when the IT band becomes irritated or inflamed due to repetitive friction with the underlying bone, often causing pain on the outer part of the knee.

The primary functions of the IT band include:

- The IT band stabilizes the hip and knee joints during movements like walking, running, and standing. It helps prevent excessive sideways movement of the knee joint.

- The IT band assists in hip abduction, which is the movement of the leg away from the body's midline. This is important for maintaining balance and stability while walking or standing on one leg.

- During running, the IT band works with other muscles and structures to control leg movement and provide stability.

- The IT band plays a role in decelerating the leg during activities like running and walking, helping to control the impact forces on the knee joint.

Causes of Iliotibial Band Syndrome:

- Engaging in repetitive movements involving frequent knee bending and straightening, such as running, cycling, hiking, or prolonged downhill activities.

- Muscle imbalances and tightness in the hip, thigh, and gluteal muscles cause increased tension in the iliotibial band. Weak hip abductors or tight hip flexors can alter hip and knee mechanics, leading to more friction on the IT band.

- Rapidly increasing physical activity intensity, duration, or frequency without sufficient adaptation time, results in excessive strain on the iliotibial band.

- Certain anatomical factors, like a naturally tight iliotibial band or abnormal hip or knee alignment, make individuals more susceptible to ITBS.

- Wearing worn-out or unsuitable footwear lacking proper support potentially affects lower limb alignment and contributes to ITBS.

Symptoms associated with ITBS:

- The main symptom is pain on the outer side of the knee, usually just above the joint line. The pain may feel as sharp, stabbing, or burning sensation. Pain may intensify when descending stairs or running downhill, as the iliotibial band rubs more intensely against the lateral part of the knee joint.

- Discomfort increases during activities that require knee bending and straightening, such as running, cycling, hiking, or climbing stairs.

- In some cases, there may be mild swelling on the outer side (lateral aspect) of the knee due to inflammation in the affected area.

- Palpating the outer knee area may reveal tenderness and discomfort.

- Some patients may experience a popping or snapping sensation when the iliotibial band moves over the lateral knee joint.

- The knee may feel stiff, especially after rest or in the morning.

- Discomfort may persist after physical activities, and in some cases, it can interfere with daily activities or rest.

The severity of ITBS symptoms can vary from person to person. While some patients may experience mild discomfort that improves with rest, others may have more persistent and intense pain that affects their ability to engage in sports or physical activities.

Sports commonly associated with an increased risk of developing ITBS include:

- Long-distance running, such as marathon running, and even short-distance sprints can lead to ITBS due to the repetitive nature of the knee movements during running.

- Cycling, especially over long distances or on stationary bikes, can result in ITBS due to the continuous knee bending and straightening involved in pedalling.

- Hiking on uneven terrain or participating in trail running, mainly downhill, can increase the risk of ITBS due to altered lower limb mechanics and increased stress on the iliotibial band.

- Soccer involves frequent direction changes, cutting, and running, which can contribute to ITBS, especially in players with muscle imbalances or inadequate warm-up routines.

- In basketball, sudden stopping, starting, and lateral movements can stress the iliotibial band and lead to ITBS, particularly if players have weak hip abductor muscles.

- Rowers can be at risk of ITBS due to the repetitive bending and straightening of the knees during rowing strokes.

- Tennis players, especially those who play on hard surfaces, can experience ITBS due to the repetitive knee movements involved in running and hitting the ball.

While the exact prevalence can vary depending on the specific population studied and the definition used for diagnosing ITBS, it's estimated that ITBS is the second most common cause of knee pain due to overuse after patellofemoral dysfunction.

Lower Leg Injuries

Shin Splints

Shin splints, also known as medial tibial stress syndrome (MTSS), is a common condition characterized by pain along the medial edge of the tibia. It is often caused by repetitive stress on the muscles, tendons, and bones in the lower leg, typically occurring during activities that involve running, jumping, or dancing. Shin splints are frequently seen in athletes, especially runners and individuals who engage in high-impact activities.[4] Shin splints primarily involve the tibia, tibialis posterior and tibialis anterior and their tendons.

The primary symptom is pain along the medial or inner edge of the tibia, usually over a broad area. The pain is often described as a dull, aching sensation and may worsen during physical activities. The pain may be more noticeable during rest or at night.

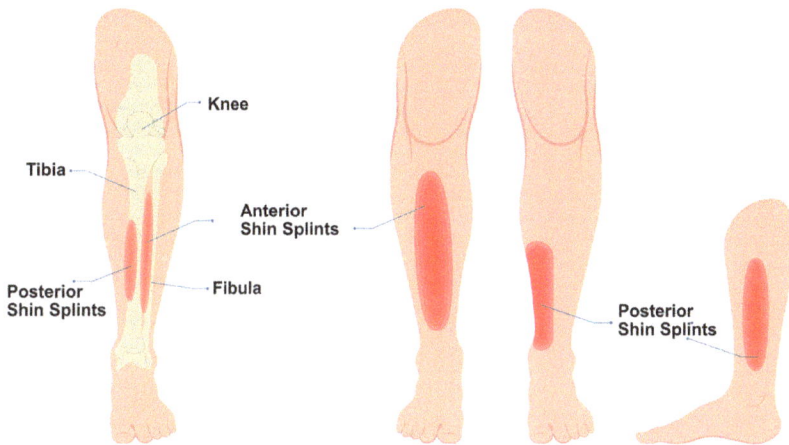

Medial Tibial Stress Syndrome

Causes of Shin Splints

The exact cause of shin splints is unclear; however, the risk factors are related to overuse or excessive stress on the lower leg. Factors that can contribute to the development of shin splints include:

- Activities involving repetitive impact on hard surfaces, such as running or jumping, can strain the lower leg structures.

- Rapidly increasing the intensity or duration of physical activities without adequate conditioning can lead to shin splints.

- Poor biomechanics and abnormalities in foot arches, gait, or lower limb alignment can contribute to excessive stress on the shin.

- Wearing improper or worn-out footwear that lacks sufficient cushioning and support can exacerbate shin splints.

- Training on hard or uneven surfaces may increase the risk of shin splints.

The reader should note that the condition described above differs from compartmental syndrome. Compartment syndrome is a serious medical condition involving increased pressure within a muscle compartment, leading to reduced blood flow and potential damage to nerves and muscles. Compartment syndrome is a medical emergency and immediate treatment is necessary to prevent permanent damage. The pain with the compartmental syndrome is intense and out of proportion to the injury or activity. The pain may feel deep and throbbing. Other symptoms may include numbness or tingling sensation due to the nerves and skin discolouration, which may appear pale and dusky due to reduced blood supply.

Calf Strain

A calf strain, also known as a calf muscle strain or pulled muscle, is an injury that occurs when the gastrocnemius and soleus muscle in the back of the lower leg are stretched or torn. Calf strains can range in severity from mild (grade I), moderate strain (grade II) to severe (grade III). Common causes of calf strains include sudden or excessive force on the calf muscles, such as during explosive movements in sports like sprinting or jumping, or when there is a rapid change in direction. Overuse, muscle fatigue, or inadequate warm-up and stretching can also contribute to calf strains.

Symptoms of a calf strain typically include:

- Pain or a sudden sharp sensation in the calf.

- Swelling and bruising in the affected area.

- Weakness or difficulty in using the calf muscles.

- Tenderness when touching the calf.

- In more severe cases, a popping or snapping sensation may be felt or heard at the time of the injury.

Common Causes of Calf Strains:

- Sudden or excessive force, such as sprinting, jumping, or changing direction abruptly. This often happens in sports like basketball, soccer, track and field, and tennis.

- Failing to properly warm up before physical activity. Cold muscles are less flexible and more prone to injury.

- Repetitive movements, especially if performed without adequate rest and recovery.

- When the calf muscles become fatigued during intense or prolonged exercise, the risk of strain increases because fatigued muscles do not provide support and stability.

- Dehydration and electrolyte imbalances can lead to muscle cramps, including in the calves.

TCM Treatment of Knee

As discussed previously, acupuncture treatment for an acute knee condition, that is during the first seventy-two hours is not advised as inserting acupuncture needle at the site of an injury can exacerbate the inflammatory response. Needling an injured area can also be painful. It is also unlikely that a TCM practitioner will come across acute injuries. However, if treatment is to be carried out during acute injuries, points (not local or adjacent) should be chosen that alleviate pain and promote reduce inflammation. During this stage the primary goals are to manage pain, reduce swelling and inflammation, and promote the initial stages of healing. Acute points such as LI4, SP6, GB34 and ST36 and auricular points are useful (as long as they are not at the site of the injury). As with other acute injuries, PRICE: protection, rest, ice, cold and elevation is used to manage the (acute) condition

During the subacute stage, which follows the acute stage, the objective is to *relieve pain, clear Heat, resolve toxins and dispel local stasis and so promote healing*. Treatment during the subacute phase will depend on the severity of the injury and the presenting symptoms. Local, adjacent, distal, and Ashi points are used. If swelling is still present around the area, needling local points is not advised as this may cause a further inflammatory response, and the resulting swelling will delay healing. Adjacent, distal points and Ashi points can be used instead.

During the early phase of a subacute injury, the points needled are manipulated strongly. In contrast, in the late subacute phase, which may be several weeks after the initial injury or when treating chronic injuries, the points are not manipulated, or if needled, only light manipulation is applied. The author's preference is to use light manipulation.

Local and Adjacent Points

Please see Appendix 1 for Acupuncture Point Location.

- **GB34:** Is the meeting point of the Sinews. As the Essential Questions Chapter 17 states, "knees are the residence of the sinews when the knees cannot flex and extend.......... then the sinews are exhausted.

  GB34 is the main point for any knee problem, whether lateral, medial, or anterior, as it benefits the sinews and joints and activates the channel. This point also moderates acute knee conditions. GB34 can be helpful for conditions such as shin splints and patellar tendinopathy.

  Needling, perpendicular: 1cun to 1.5cun.

- **ST34:** Point used when treating the knee, particularly for Painful Obstruction Syndrome, Damp, Wind, and Cold.

The point is located above the knee, so it is an excellent adjacent point for a painful knee, particularly in acute conditions.

If the knee is stiff (in addition to being painful), ST34 can be combined with SP10, GB34, and SP9.

Needling, perpendicular: 1cun to 1.5cun.

- **Xiyan** is a pair of acupuncture points located below the patella. The lateral acupoint is ST35 (Dubi) and the medial acupoint is MN-LE-16 (Nei Xiyan). ST35 is located with the knee flexed. The point is at the lower border of the patella, in the hollow below the patella and lateral to the patellar ligament.

These points should be used as a local point for treating knee disorders.

If symptoms are felt below the knee, can combine with LIV7, ST36, and GB34.

- **ST36:** Practitioners will be familiar with this point as a significant point to tonify Qi and Blood. ST 36, however, is also a beneficial local point for knee symptoms as it tonifies Zheng QI (Defensive Qi). When needled locally, it will strengthen the immune system and defend against attack from external pathogenic Wind, Damp and Cold.

Combine ST36 with ST35, LIV7, and GB34 for anterior knee symptoms.

In the early subacute stage, with redness, swelling, and pain, can combine with ST33, LIV7 and BL40.

ST36 can also be used as a distal point for anterior knee pain, such as patellar tendinopathy.

Needling: Perpendicular insertion, 1cun to 1.5cun

- **GB33:** is needled for symptoms of pain, stiffness, redness and swelling on the lateral aspect. As the Gall Bladder and Liver channels control the sinews, GB33 is used for tendon and as well as ligament injuries. As the point relaxes the sinews, GB33 can also be used for subacute conditions. GB33 is also a valuable point for symptoms of Tensor Fascia Latae and knee where it takes its attachment (Tibia).

Needling, perpendicular: 1cun to 1.5cun.

- **GB35:** removes obstruction from the channel, and so stops pain. It also relaxes the sinews. The point can be used during the subacute stage for symptoms such as cramps, swelling, and stiffness of the leg muscles.

Needling, perpendicular: 1cun to 1.5cun.

- **SP6:** is another valuable local point for leg pain, especially along the Spleen channel. SP6 also moves Blood and eliminates stasis, alleviating pain locally and along the pathway. SP 6 is also the meeting point of the Spleen, Liver, and Kidney; it can be used when the athlete suffers from recurring, chronic injury due to blood or yin deficiency as well as organ pathology. It can also function to resolve Dampness.

Needling, perpendicular: 1cun to 1.5cun. It is contraindicated in pregnancy.

- **LIV8:** Being just distal to patella, this point can be used for knee joint point, patella tendinopathy, and injury to the medial collateral ligaments (both acute and chronic), as it also relaxes the sinews. In an acute injury, after inserting the needle, the athlete is asked to move the lower leg gently to ease the pain and the stiffness (with the needle inserted).

Needling, perpendicular: 1cun to 1.5cun.

- **LIV7:** A local point for symptoms affecting the knee and the pain of the medial aspect of the leg. Being just posterior, approximately one cun to the location of SP9, LIV 7 is sometimes confused with SP9, especially if the knee is painful. To avoid this, locate SP 9 (posterior border of the tibia) first, then 1cun posterior to this is LIV7, which on pressure will feel sensitive.

Needling, perpendicular: 1cun to 1.5cun.

The posterior aspect of the leg, that is, the calf muscles, is not frequently a cause of concern unless there are contributing factors causing symptoms. These factors mainly tend to be physical, such as a tight gastrocnemius, possibly due to limb length discrepancy, and the foot pronating excessively, effectively pulling on the gastrocnemius, causing tightness and pain. Acupuncture will reduce pain but not resolve the problem. Orthotics for the foot should be considered by referring the athlete to a Podiatrist. Point combinations such as GB31 and BL60 can be used for calf pain.

Distal Points

In any injury to muscles or ligaments (sinews), in addition to local points, at least one distal point must be used. Points on the opposite side can be chosen as well. As with local and adjacent points, the channel affected will guide the selection of distal points.

The meridian affected should be identified when treating knee injuries, as this determines the acupuncture points to use. For example, if the pain is along the anterior aspect of the knee, choose points on the Stomach Channel; if the pain is along the lateral aspect, then the Gall Bladder Channel and so on.

The meridians around the knee and the lower leg are:

- Gall Bladder Channel on the lateral aspect
- Bladder Channel on the posterior aspect of the leg
- Stomach Channel on the anterior aspect of the leg

- Spleen Channel on the medial aspect of the leg.

- Liver and Kidney Channels on the medial aspect of the lower leg as they ascend proximally towards the thigh.

Distal Points

- **ST41:** This Jing River point is needled 0.5cun and used as a distal point for symptoms along the Stomach Channel. ST41 is useful when the knee and ankle are affected. ST41 activates the channel and alleviates pain along the channel.

- **SP5:** Needled perpendicular: 0.2cun to 0.5cun. SP 5 is a River Point, so Qi is diverted to joints, benefitting bones and sinews. Removes obstruction, alleviating pain. Painful Obstruction point for Dampness. It can be used for symptoms on the medial side, such as Shin Splints.

- **GB40:** Needled perpendicular: 0.5cun to 1.0cun. GB40 is a Yuan Source point that activates the GB channel, alleviates pain, and is used for symptoms along the lateral aspect of the leg. If pain is also felt in the thigh and the hip, GB40 can be combined with GB30 and GB34.

- **BL60:** Needled perpendicular 0.5cun to 1cun for symptoms along the posterior aspect of the leg and higher up as the point activates the entire Bladder channel. BL 60 also relaxes the sinews.

- **LU6.** The point can be needled as an upper/lower point. The needle side will depend on whether treating an acute or chronic; for acute conditions needle the opposite side, whereas the affected side is needled for chronic injury.

Pain along Meridian

- **Bladder Channel, use;**

  BL36, BL40, BL58 and BL63. These points harmonize collaterals and alleviate pain.

- **Gall Bladder, use;**

  GB34, GB40 and GB41. Improves circulation of Qi and Blood.

- **Stomach Channel;**

  ST34, ST35, GB40 and GB41. Improves the circulation of Qi and Blood.

- **Liver Channel;**

  LIV3, LIV5, LIV6, and LR8. Harmonises collaterals and helps with Stagnation.

- **Kidney Channel;**

  KID3, KID4, KID5 and KID10. Strengthens Kidney (related to knee) and regulates Qi and Blood.

- **Spleen Channel;**

  SP3, SP4 and SP10. Strengthens Spleen and regulates Qi and Blood.

Painful Obstruction Syndrome (POS) as a cause of Knee Pain

POS is the cause of knee pain when there is a weakness of Wei or Defensive Qi and pathogens invade the body. When the skin pores fail to open and close properly, external pathogenic factors can invade the body and knees, causing the flow of Qi and Blood to slow down or stagnate so that knee pain results and joint movements, such as flexion and extension, are also limited. The clinical symptoms will vary according to the different pathogenic factors.

Depending on symptoms and the pathogens, can use the general Adjunct points below. These points would be used with local, adjacent and Ashi points.

- *Wind Bi* – BL 12, BL 17, SP 10 or DU 16; points which promote Blood and so eliminate Wind.

- *Cold Bi* – BL 23, CV 4 or Ren 4. Warms Kidney strengthens Yang, and so eliminates Cold.

- *Damp Bi* – SP 6, SP 9, GB 34 or ST 36 strengthens Spleen and eliminates Dampness.

A useful technique for needling muscle Bi (exterior or interior) is using "Triple puncture". Insert one needle to the depth of the muscle affected and in the centre of the muscle and insert two needles bilaterally to either side of the previous needle.

If needling for Tendon Bi, insert a needle near an affected tendon, combining with GB 34.

The main difference between muscle and tendon BI is that muscle Bi has more soreness, whereas the area will feel stiff with tendon Bi. However, it may be challenging to differentiate between the two types of Bi.

Chronic Knee Pain

Chronic knee pain can be caused by various underlying patterns of disharmony. As TCM views the body holistically, chronic knee pain can be considered as a manifestation of these imbalances in the body's Qi, Blood circulation, and organ imbalance.

Common patterns that may be associated with chronic knee pain in TCM include:

- Qi and Blood Stagnation can lead to chronic knee pain. This pattern is often associated with injuries, overuse, or prolonged inactivity that disrupts the flow of Qi and Blood in the knee joint.

- Dampness and Phlegm accumulation are pathogenic factors affecting the knee. When these accumulate in the knee joint, they can lead to heaviness, swelling, and aching pain. This pattern is often seen in individuals with conditions like osteoarthritis.

- External factors like Wind, Cold, and Dampness can penetrate the body and affect the joints, including the knees. This pattern can lead to acute or chronic knee pain, often worsening in damp or cold weather.

- Kidneys play a vital role in supporting the lower body, including the knees. Kidney deficiency, either in Yin or Yang aspects, can lead to chronic knee pain and instability. It may also be associated with lower backache.

- Emotions and stress can affect the Liver in TCM, leading to Liver Qi stagnation. This pattern is often associated with chronic knee pain, especially when it is triggered or worsened by emotional stress.

- Blockages or disruptions in the meridians can lead to chronic knee pain.

- Imbalances in Yin and Yang energies in the body can affect the knees. For example, Yin deficiency can lead to dryness and heat in the knees, while Yang deficiency can result in coldness and weakness.

Beneficial points for chronic knee pain:

The selection and combination of points depend on the individual's specific symptoms, underlying imbalances and presenting syndromes. Some of the points which may be beneficial for chronic knee pain include.

Local Points around the Knee:

- **Xiyan** (Extra Point): Positioned just below the patella, Xiyan is effective for knee pain, stiffness, and reduced range of motion. It's particularly useful for addressing local swelling and discomfort.

- **EX-LE4** (Neixiyan): Positioned inside the knee joint crease, used for knee pain, swelling, and stiffness.

- **SP9:** Benefits knee pain, stiffness, and swelling. It is associated with strengthening the Spleen and regulating water metabolism, which is often relevant in knee issues.

- **SP11:** Beneficial for knee pain, swelling, and promoting circulation in the area.

- **ST34:** A commonly used point for knee symptoms, including pain, swelling, and weakness. It helps in regulating the flow of Qi and Blood in the knee area.

Meridian Points:

- **GB34:** An important point in treating knee pain, addressing stiffness, and strengthening tendons and ligaments around the knee.

- **GB39:** Beneficial for knee pain, swelling, and stiffness. It's linked to promoting the flow of Qi and Blood in the lower extremities.

- **SP10:** Connected with Blood Stasis and related conditions and is used for managing knee pain, especially in cases where Blood stasis is a contributing factor.

- **ST36:** Often used for overall pain management, strengthening the body, and improving flow of Qi through the legs.

Distal Points:

- **LI4 and LIV3:** These points are often utilized to address pain and promote overall balance in the body. While not directly related to the knee, they can help in regulating Qi and reducing pain perception.

- **KID3:** Used for strengthening the Kidneys and benefitting knee when symptoms related to Kidney Qi deficiency.

- **BL60:** Useful point for addressing lower back pain, leg pain, and knee issues related to Qi and Blood stagnation.
- Ah Shi points can also be used

Conclusion

Traditional Chinese Medicine offers a holistic approach to the treatment of knee injuries. The selection of acupuncture points in TCM is guided by an individualized assessment (according to syndrome pattern) of the patient's condition, including the underlying pattern of disharmony. Acupuncture can effectively address various factors contributing to knee problems, such as Qi and Blood Stagnation, Dampness, Wind, Cold, and imbalances in the meridians.

Acupuncture points like GB30, GB34, ST36, and SP6 are commonly utilized to target knee pain and promote circulation, alleviating discomfort and supporting the body's natural healing processes. Additionally, Ashi points and local points near the knee area may be employed to address pain and inflammation directly.

References

1. www.aafp.org/pubs/afp/issues/2010.
2. www:cks.nice.org.uk/topics/knee-pain-assessment/diagnosis/examination.
3. www.jospt.org/doi/10.2519.
4. www.nidirect.gov.uk/conditions/shin-splints.

Chapter 16

The Foot Anatomy, Injuries and TCM Treatment

The primary function of the foot is to provide support and bear the weight of the body during activities like standing, walking and running. Additionally, the foot acts as a natural shock absorber, cushioning the impact forces generated when the foot meets the ground, protecting the body from uneven upward stress. Equally essential is the role of the foot in maintaining balance and stability, which is due to its muscles and ligaments adapting to various terrains. Sensory receptors in the foot provide feedback about the environment's texture and temperature, crucial for balance and adapting to different surfaces.

The Foot Anatomy

- Despite the size of the foot, the anatomy of the foot is intricate and complex. The foot comprises a total of twenty-six bones, including seven tarsal bones, five metatarsal bones, and phalanges. These bones interact, not only providing the necessary rigidity for weight-bearing and stability but also allowing for a broad range of movements and acting as mobile adapter for various surfaces.

- The foot also has a multitude of joints, including the essential ankle joint, subtalar joint, and various metatarsophalangeal and interphalangeal joints. These joints serve the dual purpose of giving stability and enabling the flexibility required for the movements involved in activities such as walking and running.

- The complexity of the foot also extends to its muscular arrangement, having both intrinsic and extrinsic muscles, all of which work together in a coordinated manner. The extrinsic muscles, like the tibialis anterior and gastrocnemius have been discussed previously. The numerous intrinsic muscles are beyond the scope of this book.

Foot Arches

There are three curved arches of the foot formed by the arrangement of bones, ligaments, tendons, and fascia in the sole of the foot. The three arches of the foot are:

- **Medial Longitudinal Arch**: This is the most prominent and easily visible arch of the foot. It runs along the inner edge or medial aspect of the foot and is often referred to as the "instep." The medial longitudinal arch acts as a shock absorber during activities like walking and running, helping to distribute the forces generated by body weight evenly across the foot. It is also important for maintaining balance and stability.

- **Lateral Longitudinal Arch**: This arch runs along the outer or lateral aspect of the foot. Though it is not as prominent or pronounced as the medial longitudinal arch, nevertheless the lateral longitudinal arch contributes to the foot's stability and helps with weight distribution.

- **Transverse Arch**: Spans the width of the foot and adds rigidity to the foot, allowing it to bear weight effectively and maintain its shape when the foot is in a weight-bearing position.

At the bottom of the foot is the plantar fascia, a thick, fibrous band of connective tissue running longitudinally from the calcaneus to the base of the toes. It forms what can be thought of as fourth arch of the foot. The plantar fascia maintains the arches of the foot and provides stability during various weight-bearing activities such as walking, running, and standing. Inflammation or irritation of the plantar fascia is a common cause of heel pain and is known as plantar fasciitis.

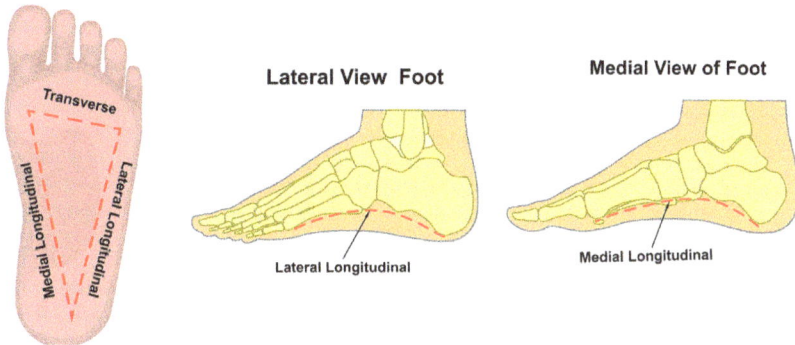

Arches of the Foot

Two Common Injuries of the Foot are:

1. Ankle Sprains

There are two types of sprains which occur at the ankle joint;

a) **An inversion or lateral sprain:** Occurs when the foot rolls inward, causing the stretching or tearing of the outer ankle ligaments. This type of ankle sprain is the most common. This is attributed to the anatomy and mechanics of the ankle joint. The relatively weaker nature of the supporting ligaments on the lateral side makes them more susceptible to sprains. The ligaments affected are the anterior talofibular ligament, calcaneofibular ligament, and posterior talofibular ligament. They are particularly prone to injury when the foot undergoes inversion, a frequent occurrence during sports and activities involving sudden changes in direction, jumping, or landing on uneven surfaces. Additionally, athletes often tend to land or plant their feet in positions that exert excessive stress on the lateral ligaments, further increasing the risk of lateral ankle sprains.

b) **Eversion or medial sprains**: Less common compared to inversion sprains. The reason for this difference is primarily related to the anatomy of the ankle joint and the way people typically move during various activities. Also, eversion sprains, require the foot to roll outward, which is a less typical movement for the ankle joint. Furthermore, the presence of the strong deltoid ligament, on the medial aspect, prevents an eversion injury. Eversion of the foot is less frequently encountered in sports and everyday activities. Eversion sprains often occur during specific situations, such as forceful outward movements of the foot or when the foot gets caught in an awkward position. The primary ligament involved in eversion sprains is the deltoid ligament.

TCM Treatment of the Sprained Ankle

In TCM the occurrence of a physical injury, such as a sprain or trauma, disrupts the harmonious flow of Qi and Blood within the body. This manifests as imbalances; Qi stagnation, where the normal Qi flow becomes obstructed, resulting in discomfort and tension. As Qi stagnates, Blood stagnates causing the accumulation of Blood in the injured area, causing swelling, bruising, pain and heat, typical signs of and inflammation. During the first seventy-two hours of an acute injury, it is not advisable to directly needle the injured area, as this can exacerbate the inflammatory response and also be painful. However, using "PRICE": Protect, Rest, Ice, Compression and Elevation is the accepted treatment during the acute stage. Once the acute phase becomes subacute, local and adjacent points can be used.

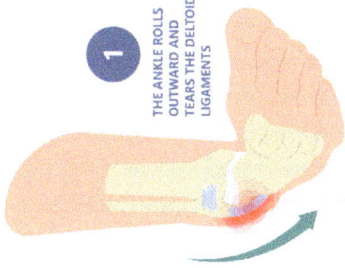

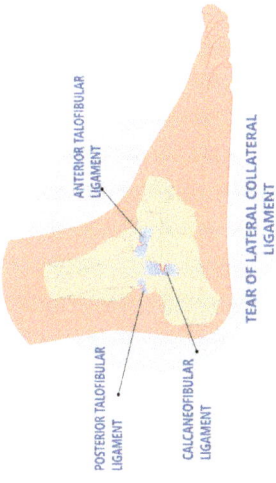

Ankle Sprains

INVERSION ANKLE SPRAINS

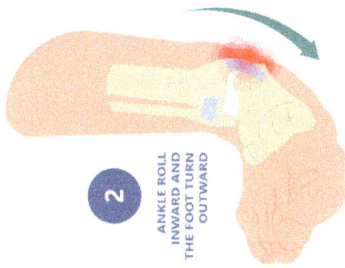

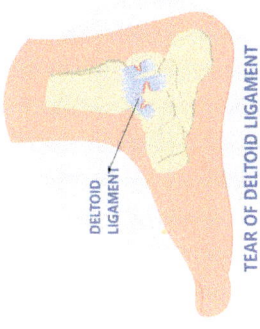

EVERSION ANKLE SPRAINS

THE ANKLE ROLLS OUTWARD AND TEARS THE DELTOID LIGAMENTS

ANTERIOR TALOFIBULAR LIGAMENT

POSTERIOR TALOFIBULAR LIGAMENT

CALCANEOFIBULAR LIGAMENT

TEAR OF LATERAL COLLATERAL LIGAMENT

ANKLE ROLL INWARD AND THE FOOT TURN OUTWARD

DELTOID LIGAMENT

TEAR OF DELTOID LIGAMENT

Subacute Treatment

The subacute phase follows an acute stage and can last for several weeks after the initial injury; the aim of the treatment is to *relieve pain, clear heat, resolve toxins, and dispel local stasis.*

During the early phase of a subacute injury, the points which are needled are manipulated strongly, whereas in the late subacute phase, which may be several weeks after the initial or when treating chronic injuries, the points are not needled at all or if needled than only light manipulation is applied.

Local and Adjacent Points

Please see Appendix 1 for Acupuncture Point Location.

Local points are chosen because of their vicinity to the symptoms and to reduce inflammation, ease painful symptoms and improve Qi and Blood circulation (remember, local points stimulate the production of pain-relieving chemicals and cause vasodilation and vascular permeability, all promoting healing).

Adjacent points are chosen due to their proximity to the injured area or clinical significance.

The local and adjacent points which can be used are:

- **GB40:** Benefits the joints and alleviates pain locally. Clears channel "opening" the foot, helping with local swelling and cramping sensation. Also, useful point when the ankle is affected by Painful Obstruction Syndrome.

  Needling: Perpendicular insertion 0.5cun to 1cun.

  If pain is felt in the heel can combine with GB39 and BL60.

- **GB41:** Used when there is pain and swelling on the dorsum of the foot or lateral ankle sprains. GB41 is also used if the injury has caused the toes to go into spasm (spastic pain).

  Needling: Perpendicular insertion 0.3cun to 0.5cun.

- **BL63:** This accumulation point is helpful in acute conditions for the relief of pain. The point also relaxes sinews, invigorates the collaterals, and activates the Channel to clear local stagnation.

  Needling: Perpendicular insertion 0.3cun to 0.5cun.

- **BL58:** Removes obstruction from the Channel, clearing stagnation and so relieves pain. The stagnation results from the injury and disruption to the flow of Qi and Blood. The point also relaxes the sinews. An excellent point to use for Achilles tendinopathy. A disorder that can cause pain, stiffness, swelling and weakness of the Achilles tendon. An alternative to BL58, BL57, can also be used.

  Needling: Perpendicular insertion 0.3cun to 0.5cun.

- **GB 34:** Has already been discussed previously. GB 34 is used for foot and ankle pain as its use benefits sinews, especially if muscles and joints are tight.

- **SP5:** A point that can be used for pain of soft tissue around the ankle as it benefits the sinews and the joint.

  Needling: Perpendicular insertion 0.2cun to 0.3cun.

- **ST41:** Activates Channel, removes obstruction, and so stops pain. It benefits the ankle as well as the lower leg. Useful point for ankle tenosynovitis (tibialis anterior and posterior, extensor digitorum longus and peroneal tendons on the lateral aspect).

  Needling: Perpendicular insertion 0.5cun

If ankle pain can be identified along the meridians below, which transgress the ankle, the following points can be used.

- Gall Bladder Channel, add GB42 and GB43 (promotes circulation of Qi)

- Stomach Channel, add ST41, ST42 and ST43 (promotes circulation of Qi)

- Liver Channel, add LIV 3 and LIV 4 (harmonize collaterals)

- Kidney Channel, add KID3, KID4 and KID5

- Spleen Channel, add SP4 and SP5

2) Plantar Fasciitis

This is a condition characterized by inflammation and irritation of the plantar fascia which as described above is a thick band of tissue that spans the plantar aspect of the foot. When the longitudinal plantar fascia becomes inflamed, it results in heel pain, particularly at its attachment point on the heel bone. The pain is often described as sharp and stabbing, and it tends to be most intense during the initial steps taken in the morning or after periods of rest. The discomfort can also escalate following extended periods of standing, walking, or running.

Several factors contribute to the onset of plantar fasciitis:

- Repetitive strain which can be caused by excessive walking, running, or prolonged standing over time.

- Individuals with high arches or flat feet may experience an uneven distribution of weight and pressure on the plantar fascia, heightening the risk of stress and inflammation.

- Wearing shoes which lack proper arch support or cushioning can increase the likelihood of developing plantar fasciitis.

- Tension in the calf muscles can influence foot mechanics and increase strain on the plantar fascia.

- Plantar fasciitis tends to be more prevalent in individuals aged 40 to 60.

- Excess body weight can impose additional strain on the plantar fascia, contributing to the development of the condition.

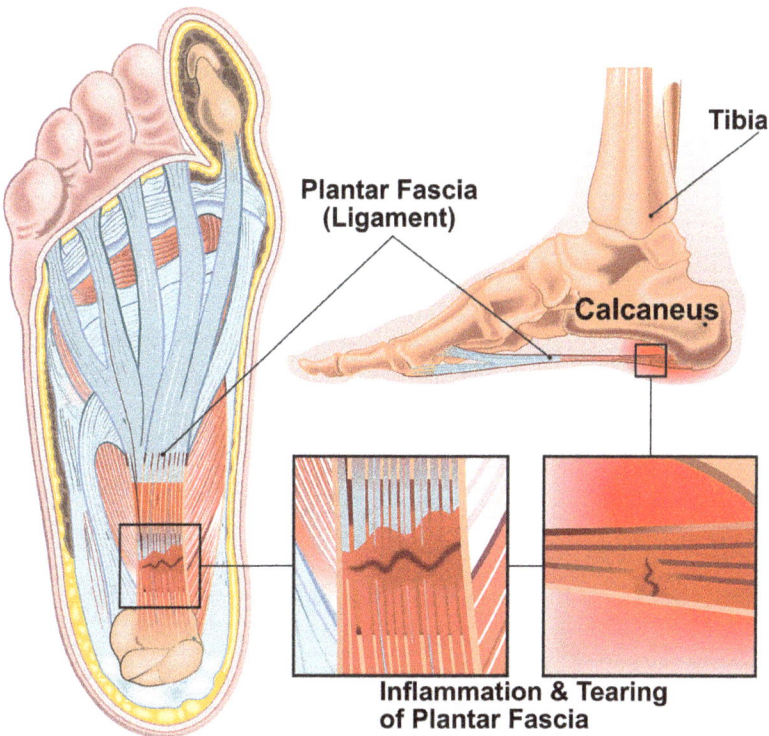

Plantar Fasciitis

TCM Treatment of Plantar Fasciitis

In Traditional Chinese Medicine, plantar fasciitis is typically due to patterns of disharmony related to the Liver, Kidney, and Spleen systems. These imbalances can lead to specific syndromes that may contribute to the development of plantar fasciitis.

Liver

In Traditional Chinese Medicine plantar fasciitis is perceived as a manifestation of an imbalance within the Liver system, which governs the smooth circulation of Qi and Blood. When the Liver becomes disrupted, it can lead to stagnation of Qi and Blood flow, consequently giving rise musculoskeletal disorders like plantar fasciitis. The stagnation of Liver Qi can obstruct the natural flow of Qi in the lower extremities, contributing to pain and inflammation in the plantar fascia. Moreover, a deficiency of Blood within the Liver system can result in inadequate nourishment of the sinews making the plantar fascia more susceptible to injury. Also, factors like external invasion of Dampness, especially when combined with Wind, may accumulate in the lower body, affecting joints, muscles, and tendons, leading to conditions like plantar fasciitis. In cases where there is an excess of Liver Yang, that is Liver Fire, inflammation and pain may arise, affecting various parts of the body, including the feet.

Kidney

An imbalance in the Kidney can contribute to the development of plantar fasciitis. As the Kidneys are regarded as vital reservoirs of Qi, essential for sustaining life, when Kidney Qi is deficient, this can lead to weakness in the bones, tendons and ligaments making them more susceptible to strain and injury, thus predisposing athletes to conditions like plantar fasciitis. Additionally, imbalances in Kidney Yin or Kidney Yang can disrupt the equilibrium necessary for the strength and integrity of tendons and ligaments, contributing to the development of plantar fasciitis. The accumulation of dampness or phlegm, can also affect the smooth flow of Qi and Blood, causing Stagnation and subsequent pain and inflammation, a common characteristic of plantar fasciitis. Furthermore, the Kidney meridian, which runs through the heel and sole of the foot, can be affected by imbalances in the Kidney system, potentially leading to discomfort or pain in these areas.

Spleen

An imbalance in the Spleen can contribute to the development of plantar fasciitis. The Spleen's vital role in transforming and transporting nutrients is important for the functioning of muscles, tendons and ligaments. When Spleen Qi is deficient, it can lead to poor digestion and absorption of nutrients, resulting in weakness in these structures including those in the feet. This can contribute to conditions like plantar fasciitis. As the Spleen also regulates fluids in the body, and if Spleen function is compromised, it can lead to the accumulation of Dampness. Excessive Dampness can impede the smooth flow of Qi and Blood, resulting in stagnation and conditions like plantar fasciitis. Also, a deficiency in Spleen Yang, responsible for providing warmth and energy, leads to reduced vitality in the muscles and tendons, increasing their susceptibility to injury.

As the Spleen meridian courses through the arches of the feet, an imbalance in the Spleen can influence the flow of Qi along this pathway, leading to discomfort or pain in the arch, a characteristic symptom of plantar fasciitis.

Blood Stagnation

Blood Stagnation can lead to localized pain, inflammation, and reduced flexibility. Stagnant Blood may accumulate in the area of the foot, exacerbating the condition.

Acupuncture Points for Plantar Fasciitis:

* Shi Mian or M-LE-5, an extra point, which is at the centre of the heel at the bottom of the foot, will move Qi and Blood. Needling: Perpendicular 0.5cun – 1cun.

- KID3 and BL60 or BL58

- KID6 and BL62

- KID4 and KID5

- KID7 and KID8

- SP6: Used to tonify Spleen Qi and promote overall circulation in the lower limbs.

- LIV3: This point is used to smooth Liver Qi and relieve pain.

- GB34: This point is commonly used to benefit the tendons and ligaments and alleviate pain.

- BL60: This point is used for pain relief in the lower limbs.

- KID1: This point is used for grounding and strengthening the Kidneys.

- Other points associated with Liver, Kidney and Spleen syndromes (as above)

Conclusion

Foot injuries are intimately linked to the anatomy of this vital part of the human body. The foot's complexity, with its numerous bones, joints, ligaments, and muscles, allows for an impressive range of movements, from walking and running to jumping and dancing. However, this complexity also makes it susceptible to a variety of injuries, such as sprains, fractures, and stress-related issues. Understanding the anatomy of the foot is useful for diagnosing, treating, and preventing these injuries effectively. Whether it's the ligaments supporting stability, the arches providing shock absorption, or the muscles enabling propulsion, each component plays a unique role in the foot's function and vulnerability to injury.

Appendix 1

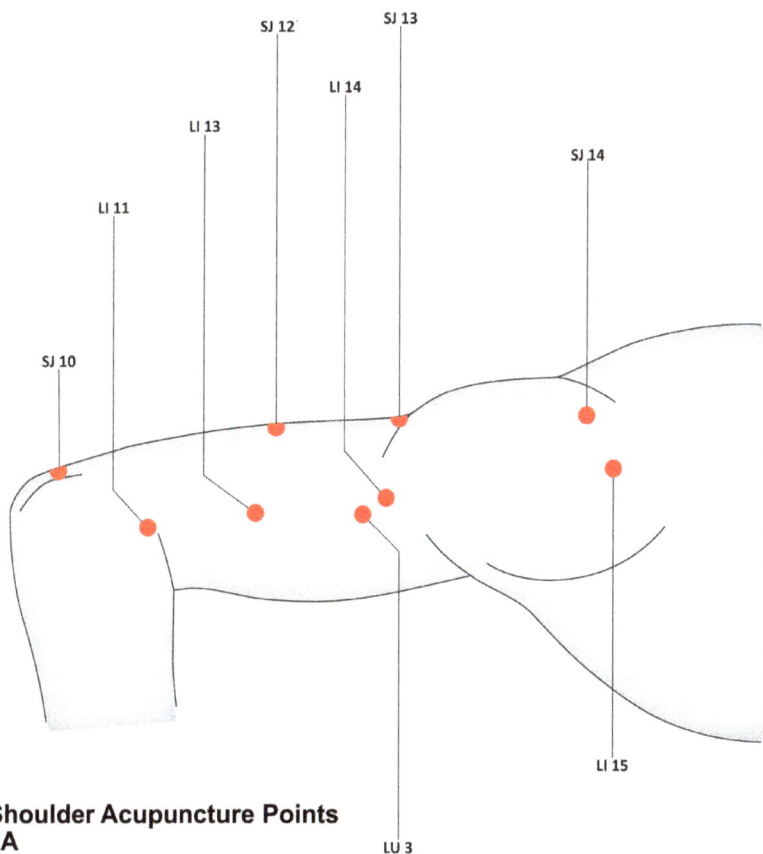

Shoulder Acupuncture Points 1A

SJ 12
SJ 13
LI 14
LI 13
SJ 14
LI 11
SJ 10
LI 15
LU 3

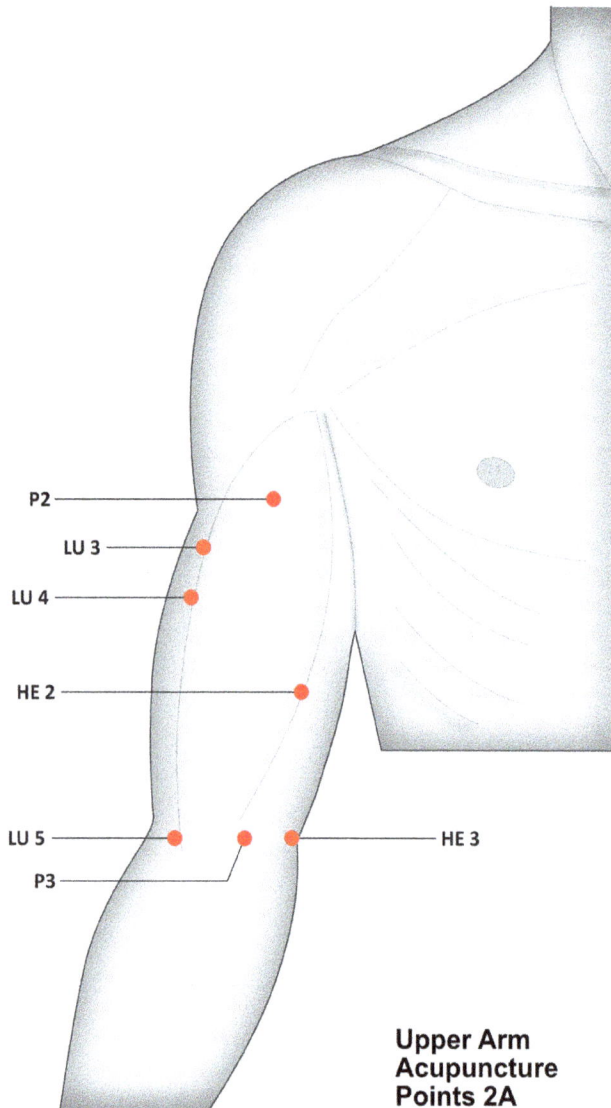

P2

LU 3

LU 4

HE 2

LU 5

P3

HE 3

**Upper Arm
Acupuncture
Points 2A**

Posterior Upper Back
Acupuncture Points 3A

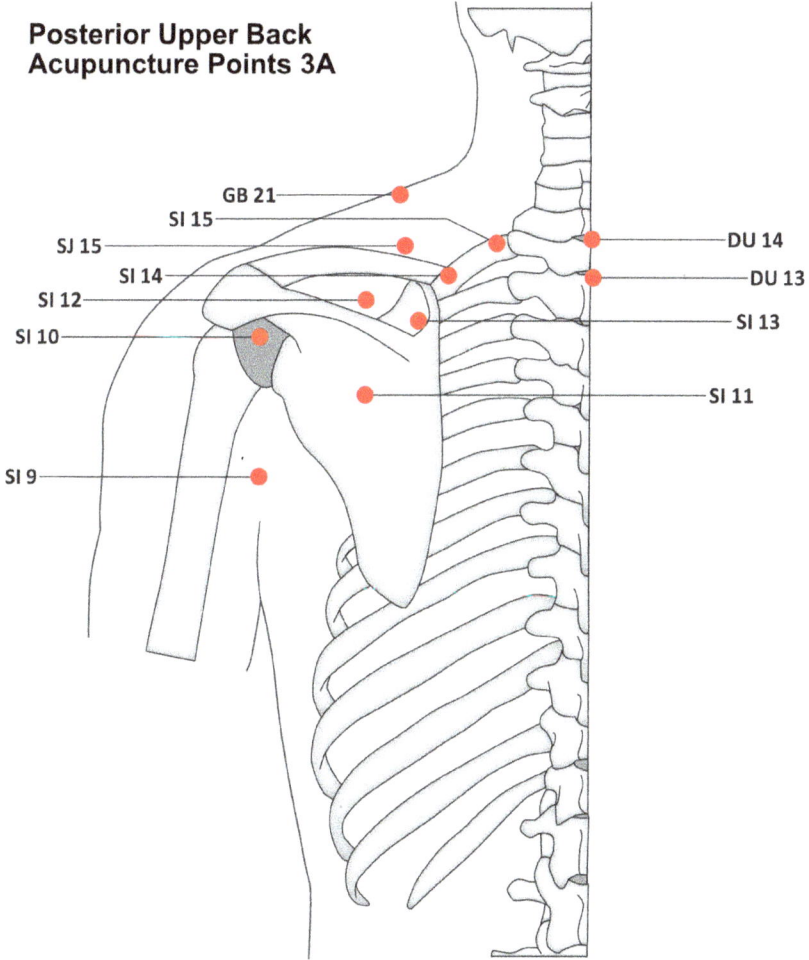

GB 21

SI 15

SJ 15

SI 14

SI 12

SI 10

SI 9

DU 14

DU 13

SI 13

SI 11

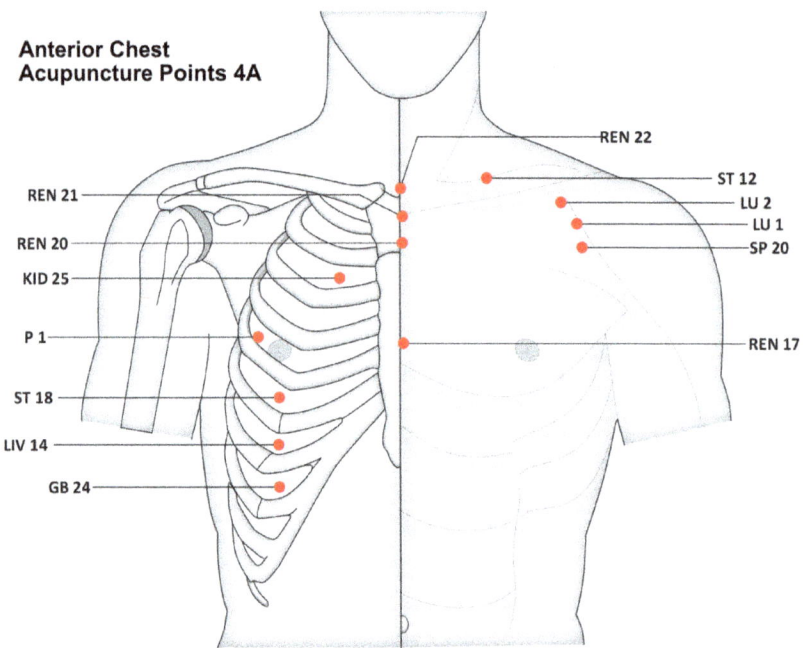

**Anterior Chest
Acupuncture Points 4A**

REN 22

ST 12

REN 21

LU 2

LU 1

REN 20

SP 20

KID 25

P 1

REN 17

ST 18

LIV 14

GB 24

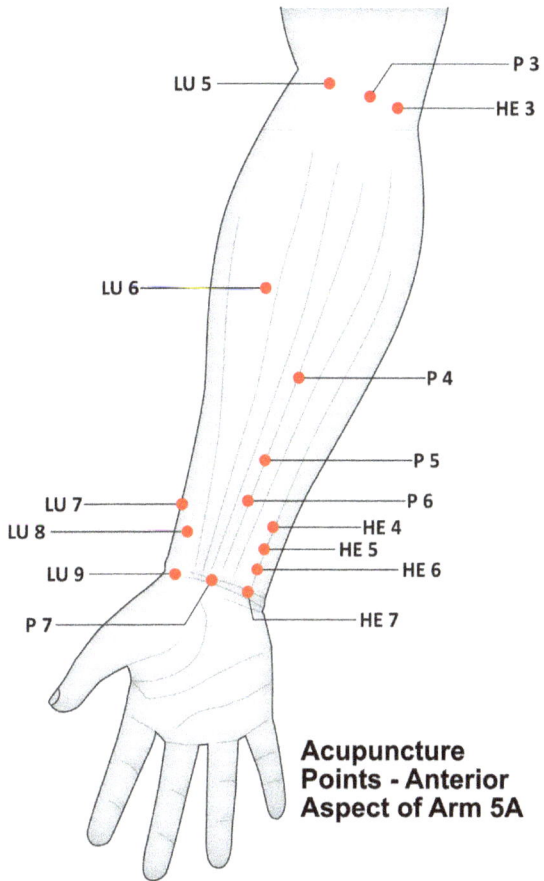

LU 5

P 3

HE 3

LU 6

P 4

P 5

LU 7

P 6

LU 8

HE 4

HE 5

LU 9

HE 6

P 7

HE 7

**Acupuncture
Points - Anterior
Aspect of Arm 5A**

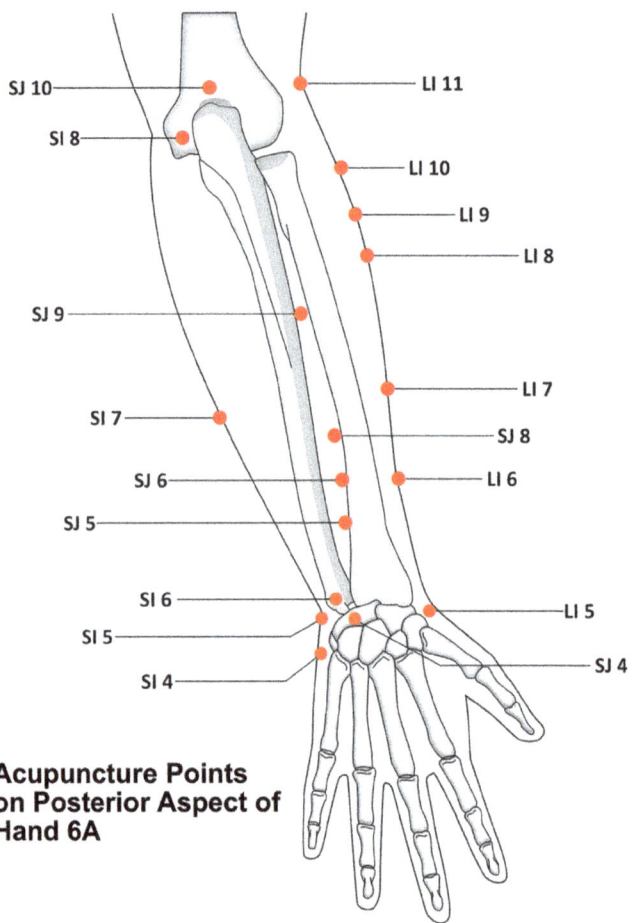

**Acupuncture Points
on Posterior Aspect of
Hand 6A**

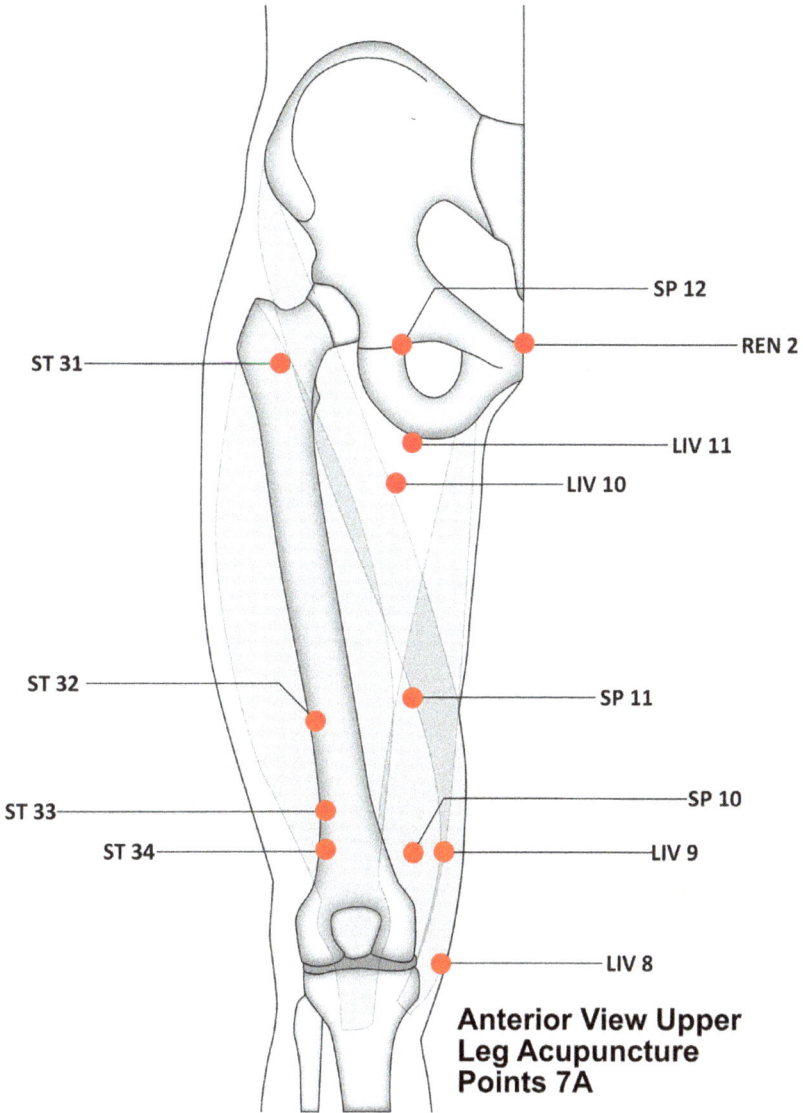

ST 31

SP 12

REN 2

LIV 11

LIV 10

ST 32

SP 11

ST 33

SP 10

ST 34

LIV 9

LIV 8

**Anterior View Upper
Leg Acupuncture
Points 7A**

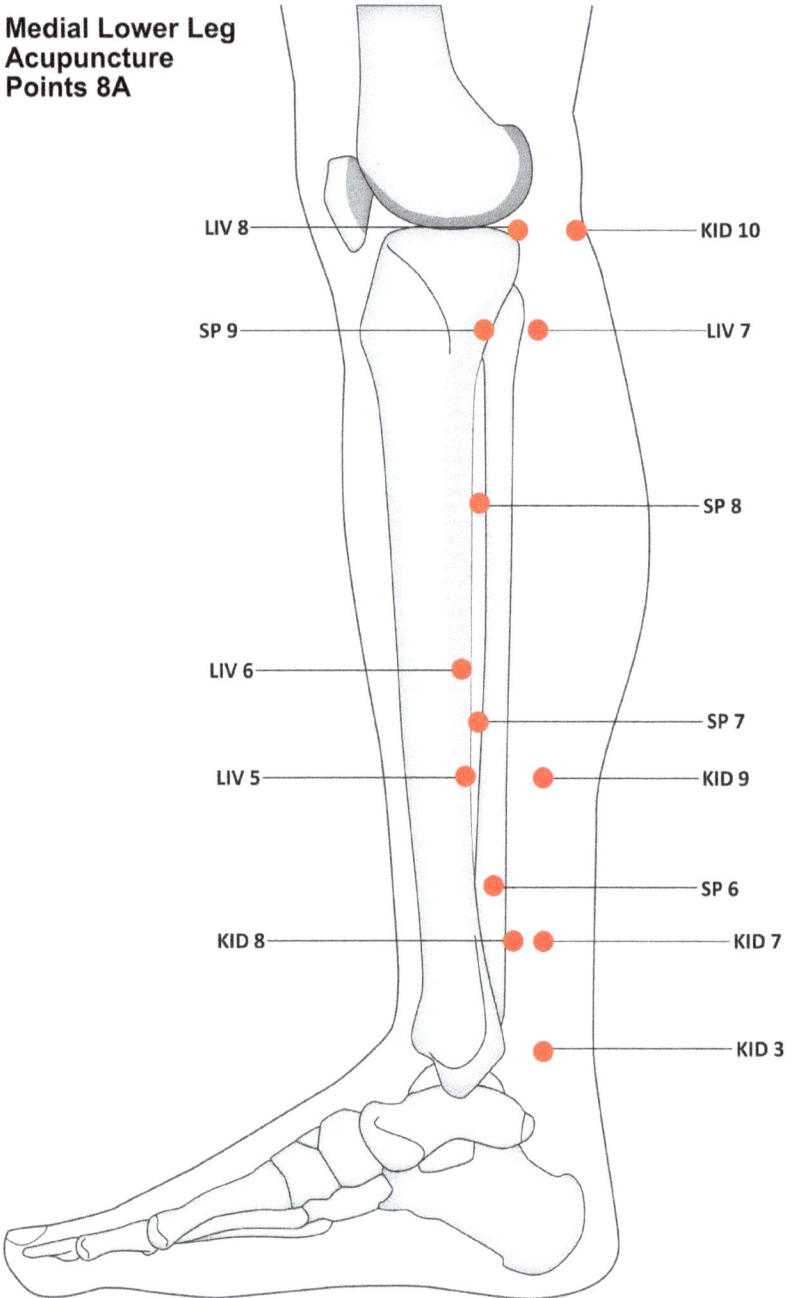

Medial Lower Leg Acupuncture Points 8A

LIV 8

KID 10

SP 9

LIV 7

SP 8

LIV 6

SP 7

LIV 5

KID 9

SP 6

KID 8

KID 7

KID 3

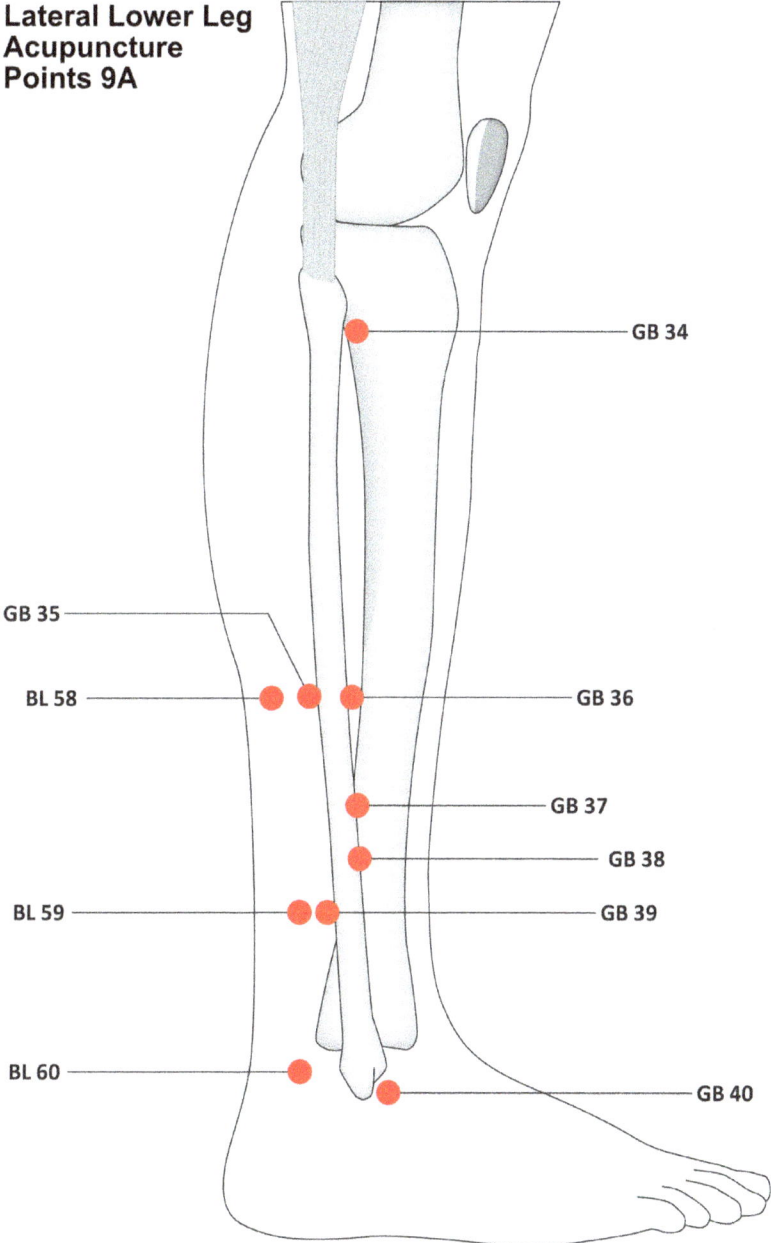

Lateral Lower Leg Acupuncture Points 9A

GB 34

GB 35

BL 58

GB 36

GB 37

GB 38

BL 59

GB 39

BL 60

GB 40

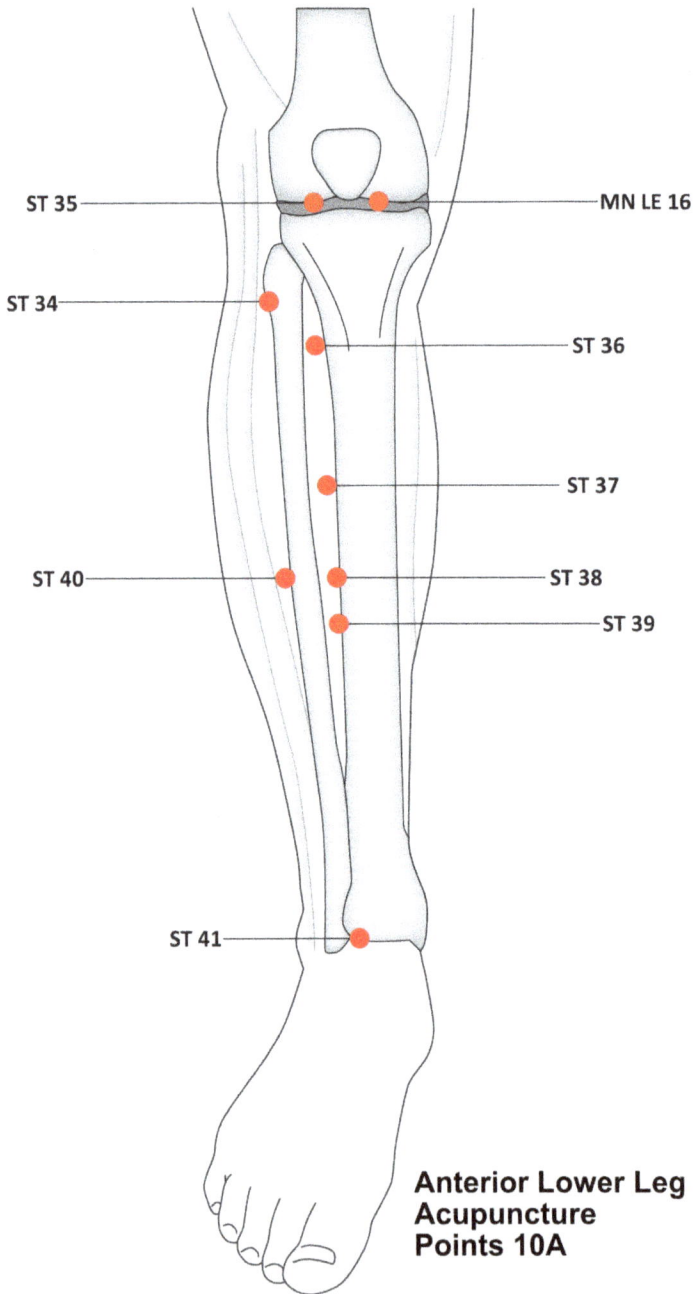

ST 35 —

MN LE 16

ST 34 —

ST 36

ST 37

ST 40 —

ST 38

ST 39

ST 41 —

**Anterior Lower Leg
Acupuncture
Points 10A**

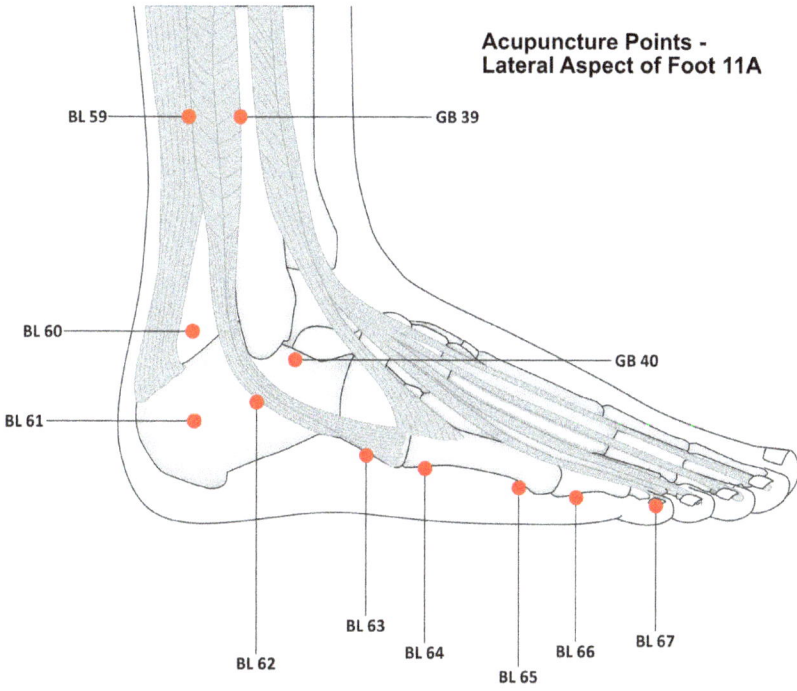

**Acupuncture Points -
Lateral Aspect of Foot 11A**

BL 59

GB 39

BL 60

GB 40

BL 61

BL 63

BL 64

BL 62

BL 66

BL 65

BL 67

Acupuncture
Points - Medial
Aspect of Foot 12A

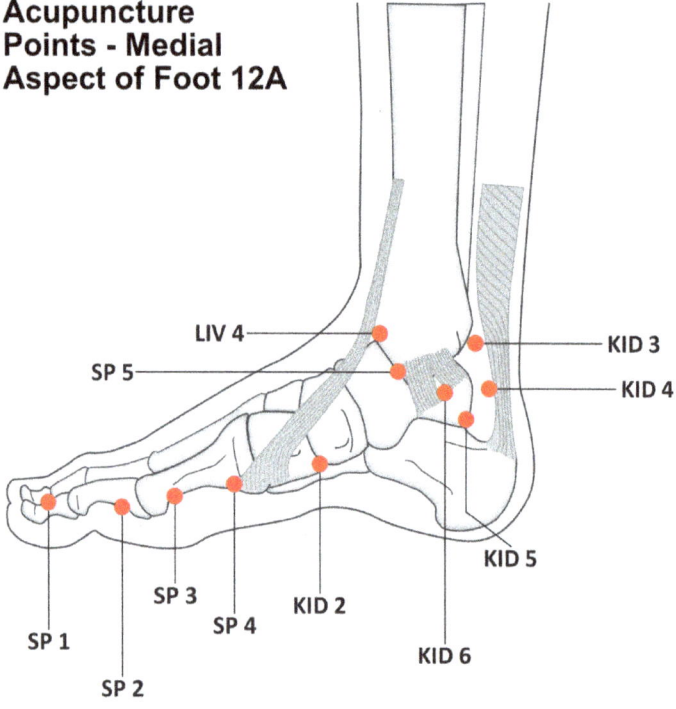

LIV 4

SP 5

KID 3

KID 4

KID 5

SP 3

KID 2

SP 4

SP 1

KID 6

SP 2

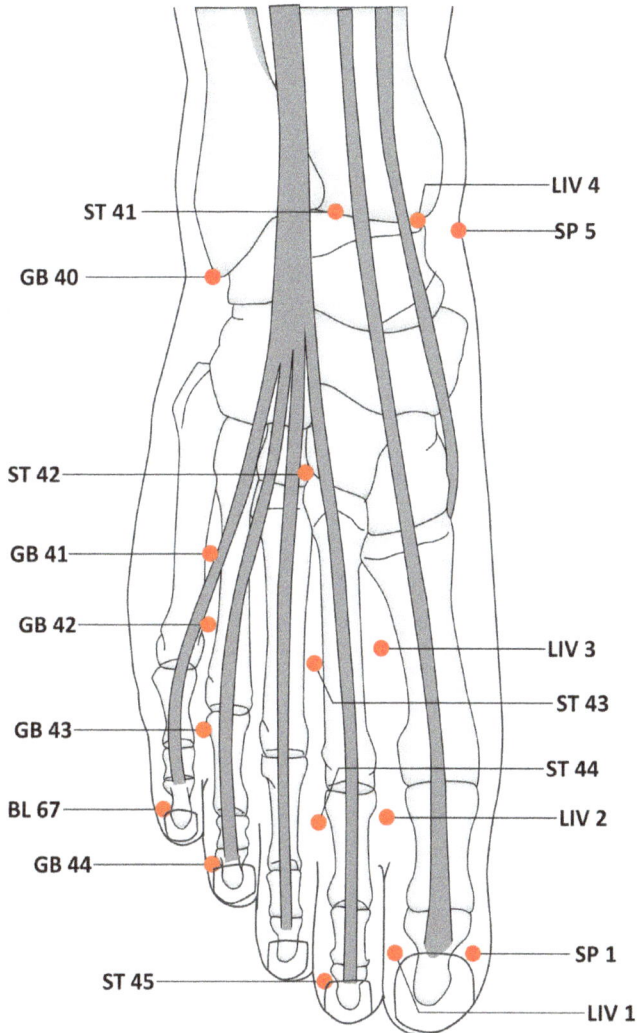

Acupuncture Points Dorsum of Foot 13A

Appendix 2

Auricular Therapy

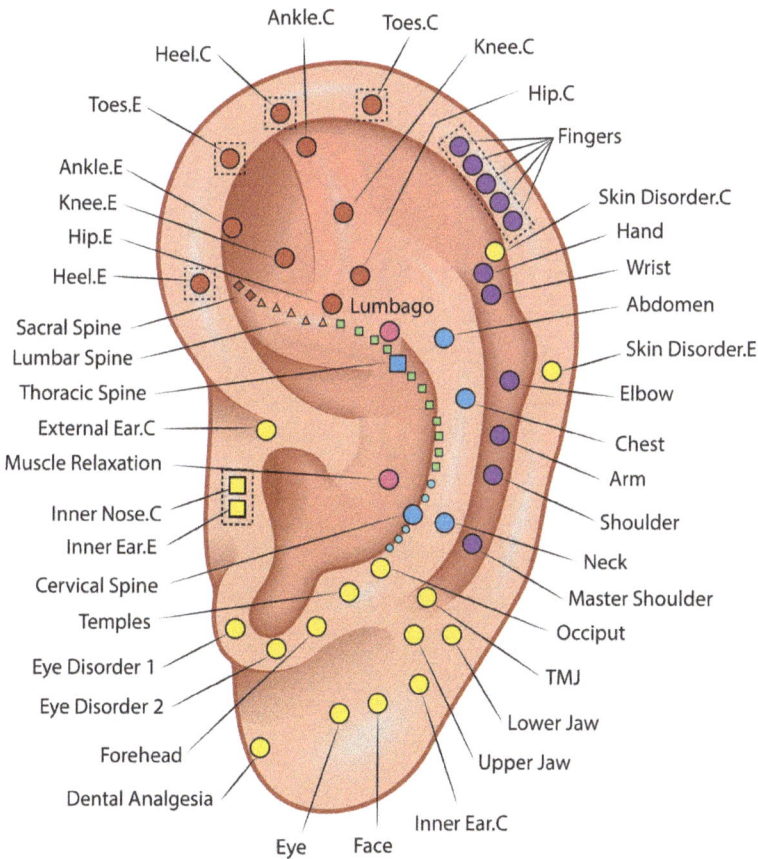

Ankle.C · Toes.C · Knee.C · Heel.C · Hip.C · Toes.E · Fingers · Ankle.E · Knee.E · Hip.E · Skin Disorder.C · Heel.E · Hand · Wrist · Lumbago · Abdomen · Sacral Spine · Skin Disorder.E · Lumbar Spine · Thoracic Spine · Elbow · External Ear.C · Chest · Muscle Relaxation · Arm · Inner Nose.C · Shoulder · Inner Ear.E · Neck · Cervical Spine · Master Shoulder · Temples · Occiput · Eye Disorder 1 · TMJ · Eye Disorder 2 · Lower Jaw · Forehead · Upper Jaw · Dental Analgesia · Inner Ear.C · Eye · Face

Appendix 3

ANATOMICAL PLANES AND SECTIONS

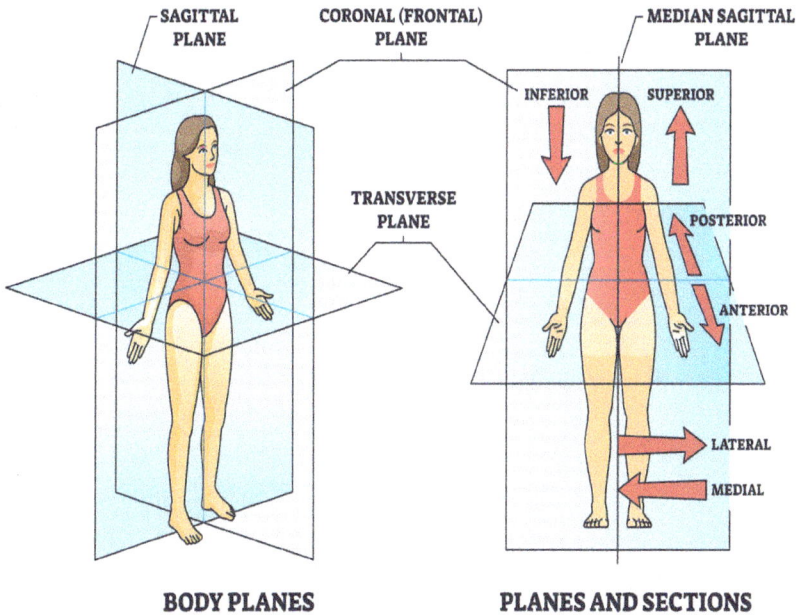

SAGITTAL PLANE

CORONAL (FRONTAL) PLANE

MEDIAN SAGITTAL PLANE

TRANSVERSE PLANE

INFERIOR

SUPERIOR

POSTERIOR

ANTERIOR

LATERAL

MEDIAL

BODY PLANES

PLANES AND SECTIONS

Index

www.ingramcontent.com/pod-product-compliance
Lightning Source LLC
Chambersburg PA
CBHW042313210326
41599CB00038B/7113

* 9 7 8 1 8 0 3 8 1 7 9 2 7 *